Contemporary Diagnosis and Management of
Sinusitis™

George A. Pankey, MD
Section on Infectious Diseases
The Ochsner Clinic, New Orleans, LA

Charles W. Gross, MD
Department of Otolaryngology, University of Virginia
Health Sciences Center, Charlottesville, VA

Michael G. Mendelsohn, MD
Department of Otolaryngology, State University
of New York Health Science Center at Brooklyn,
Brooklyn, NY

Published by Handbooks in Health Care Co.,
Newtown, Pennsylvania, USA

International Standard Book Number: 1-884065-17-1

Library of Congress Catalog Card Number: 97-71113

Contents

Introduction 5

Chapter 1   Epidemiology and Prevention 7

Chapter 2   Anatomy, Physiology,
and Pathophysiology 12

Chapter 3   Etiology 25

Chapter 4   Classification 31

Chapter 5   Diagnosis 36

Chapter 6   Imaging of the Sinuses 48

Chapter 7   Nosocomial Sinusitis, Fungal
Sinusitis, and Sinusitis in the
Immunocompromised Patient 72

Chapter 8   Antimicrobial Therapy 81

Chapter 9   Medical Therapy 91

Chapter 10   Surgical Management 106

Chapter 11   The Pediatric Patient 116

Chapter 12   Complications and Emergencies
Associated With Sinusitis 125

Chapter 13   Quality of Life 134

Index   139

This book has been prepared and is presented as a service to the medical community. The information provided reflects the knowledge, experience, and personal opinions of George A. Pankey, MD, Charles W. Gross, MD, and Michael G. Mendelsohn, MD, the principal co-authors.

Introduction

The 1993 International Conference on Sinus Disease established the following educational goals for both specialists and primary care physicians:

- Identify the patient with clinical signs and symptoms consistent with acute, recurrent acute, or chronic sinusitis.
- Recognize sinusitis as a potentially debilitating problem that requires precise diagnosis and prompt, effective treatment.
- Formulate a management plan based on what is now known about the pathophysiology of sinusitis, with special attention to the role of obstruction of the ostia and the ostiomeatal complex (OMC).
- Use a protocol for first-line medical management of acute sinusitis that includes antibiotics and decongestants as baseline therapy.
- Understand that antihistamines are indicated primarily to treat patients in whom predisposing allergic factors (release of histamines) are present.
- Predict the failure of plain x-ray films to yield conclusive information about the OMC in acute sinusitis.
- Select those patients with sinusitis who may need further evaluation by nasal endoscopy and computed tomography (CT).
- Identify patients who might benefit from appropriate referral for specialized care.
- Predict the economic and social consequences of inappropriate treatment of patients with sinusitis.

The purpose of this handbook is to help physicians who care for patients with sinusitis to become well informed about this common problem. To accomplish this goal, this book is the result of the combined efforts of an infectious disease specialist (Dr. Pankey), two otolaryngologists (Dr. Gross and Dr. Mendelsohn), and two radiologists (Jonas H. Goldstein, MD, and C. Douglas Phillips, MD).

Chapter 1

Epidemiology and Prevention

Sinusitis refers to inflammation of the mucosal lining of the nose and the paranasal sinuses. Rhinosinusitis is a more appropriate term because it is pathophysiologically more accurate. However, the traditional term, sinusitis, will be used throughout this text.

Sinusitis is the most common health-care complaint in the United States, affecting approximately 1 in 8 persons at some time in their lives. It has become the number one chronic illness for all age groups in the United States, according to the National Center for Disease Statistics. Sinusitis affects an estimated 35 million Americans each year. Its prevalence is estimated to be 5% to 15% of adults and up to 5% of children. Moreover, sinusitis continues to increase in prevalence among patients of all age groups. According to statistics, sinusitis accounted for nearly 25 million physician office visits in the United States in 1993 and 1994. Many more cases are unreported and many patients suffer without seeing a physician. Antibiotic prescriptions for sinusitis rose from 5.8 million in 1985 to 13 million in 1992. The direct medical cost of sinusitis in 1992 was $2.4 billion.

Most patients with sinusitis are treated medically by primary care physicians, although increasing numbers of patients with recurrent acute and chronic sinusitis are being treated surgically. In fact, some estimates indicate that more than 200,000 sinus surgical procedures are being performed each year in the United States. The number of patients treated surgically could decline if primary care physicians took a more aggressive medical management approach. Therefore, it is important for primary care physicians to recognize and properly diagnose acute, recurrent acute, subacute, chronic, and acute exacerbations of chronic sinusitis, especially because identifying the causes of recurrent and chronic sinusitis can be challenging. Treatment should be aimed at eliminating causative factors and controlling the inflammatory as well as the infectious components of the disease. Ideal management includes administration of preventive measures as well as the application of proper baseline medical therapy in adequate dosages and duration.

The increase in incidence of sinusitis is paralleled by enormous improvements in the past 10 years in diagnosis and treatment of sinusitis, largely because of technologic advances in nasal endoscopy and imaging, and the development of newer, more powerful antibiotics. Despite these advances, many physicians find it difficult to confirm the diagnosis of sinusitis and, as a result, too often fail to choose the ideal therapy. In fact, physicians commonly assume that patients have an allergy when they are actually suffering from an infection, or vice versa. Communication between the various disciplines is essential to the better understanding of accurate diagnosis, proper preventive measures, and appropriate therapy. As new information is acquired, it must be effectively disseminated to the primary care physicians and specialists involved in the care of patients with sinusitis.

Americans spent approximately $200 million on over-the-counter products for sinusitis in 1992, according to estimates. This represents a $50 million increase since 1989. Even though antihistamines have been shown to have only a minor role in sinusitis and upper respiratory tract infections, approximately $134 million of that $200 million was spent on products containing antihistamines. Furthermore, inappropriate choices of antibiotic, dosage, and duration are commonly made. These are prime examples of the need for better inter-disciplinary education for physicians and patients.

Although most of this book is devoted to the diagnosis and management of sinusitis, we want to emphasize the importance of prevention. Primary events in the embryology of the cranial-oral-facial region occur between the 4th and 8th weeks of fetal life. Many congenital abnormalities begin as a result of stress on the fetus in the first trimester. The sinuses must be especially sensitive because up to 50% of maxillary sinuses have incomplete septa and accessory ostia. It is well recognized that pregnant women should avoid alcohol and tobacco smoke, but more study is needed on other stresses that may have an effect on fetal sinus development. Being born without a deviated nasal septum, for example, might prevent the development of chronic sinusitis in some patients.

Obviously, upper respiratory viral infections, inhaled allergens, and irritative air pollutants (especially those that induce sneezing) are not good for the sinuses. The problem of global warming and related increased air pollution, with their likely adverse effect on the sinuses, are issues that society should address. While the avoidance of cigarette smoking is an obtainable goal, we know that smoking addiction is difficult to overcome for many patients. These factors are felt to be important in the ever-increasing incidence of sinusitis.

Vaccines are available for two of the bacterial pathogens that cause sinusitis, namely, *Streptococcus pneumoniae* and *Haemophilus influenzae* type b. The conjugated *H influenzae* type b vaccine now being used in pediatrics has clearly resulted in a dramatic decline in disease from that organism. Unfortunately, as one ages, the antibody titer from both the vaccine and exposure to *H influenzae* type b declines, so that persons over 65 years of age may not be protected. Because the population over 60 is the most rapidly growing group of patients and will make up about 20% of the population by the year 2000, studies are needed about the use of this vaccine in the elderly. Most strains of *H influenzae* associated with sinusitis are unencapsulated and untypeable. Therefore, protection may not occur after use of the available vaccine.

Sinusitis in the elderly is a common problem and, although the pneumococcal vaccine is being recommended for all individuals in this age group, less than 50% have been vaccinated. The present pneumococcal vaccine is not as effective as the conjugated ones being studied. Nevertheless, 60% to 70% of elderly persons should respond and obtain protection from 80% to 90% of the strains of *S pneumoniae* that cause respiratory disease. Therefore, it makes good sense to consider the pneumococcal vaccine as a preventive measure for all persons with any type of sinus problem. This would include those with allergy, those with anatomic defects, and those who persist in smoking.

We recommend that all patients with chronic sinus problems receive yearly influenza vaccine, pneumococcal vaccine with a booster in 5 years, and conjugated *H influenzae* type b vaccine for those 65 years of age or older. This recommendation is made despite the lack of reliable data about the efficacy of these vaccines in preventing sinusitis from the microorganisms the vaccines are directed against, or about whether cross-protection exists against untypeable strains of *H influenzae*. Research in these areas is clearly needed.

The prevention of obstruction to the flow of sinus secretions is obviously critical in preventing bacterial and fungal sinusitis. Therefore, the use of antihistamines and topical corticosteroids by nebulizers or atomizers in patients with allergic rhinitis may be effective in preventing sinusitis as well as in moderating symptoms. Obviously, avoidance of the allergen is the ideal preventive measure.

Nasal congestion secondary to colds or allergy is a relative contraindication to air travel, but many patients elect to fly anyway. The Aerospace Medical Association recommends that these patients take a systemic decongestant (with an antihistamine in allergy patients) as well as spray the nasal passages with a topical, long-acting nasal decongestant before the flight and before the descent. Air travelers with sinusitis are also advised to chew gum, swallow frequently, and learn how to perform Valsalva's maneuver to clear their ears. This maneuver is accomplished by holding the nose and gently generating pressure against the closed mouth and glottis every 30 seconds. Medical care should be available at the patient's destination in case sinusitis develops.

Many anatomic and developmental abnormalities can be surgically corrected if diagnosed and treated expeditiously, including removal of nasal polyps and nasoseptal deviations. Endoscopic surgery has allowed otolaryngologists to be more aggressive in managing nasal polyps. Early referral for endoscopic evaluation of allergic patients may prevent the development of chronic sinusitis. Proper care of the maxillary teeth and gums can be a major factor in the prevention of maxillary sinusitis because the molars are just beneath the sinus floor mucosa.

The importance of prevention is clear-cut, especially with the emergence of multiple drug-resistant bacterial pathogens, many of which cause sinusitis. If sinusitis is prevented, it is likely that many cases of bronchitis and pneumonia will be too.

Selected Readings

Giebink GS: Childhood sinusitis: pathophysiology, diagnosis and treatment. *Pediatr Infect Dis J* 1994;13:S55-S58.

Gwaltney JM Jr, Jones JG, Kennedy DW: Medical management of sinusitis: educational goals and management guidelines. The International Conference on Sinus Disease. *Ann Otol Rhinol Laryngol Suppl* 1995;167:22-30.

Kaliner MA, Osguthorpe JD, Fireman P, et al: Sinusitis: bench to bedside. Current findings, future directions. *Otolaryngol Head Neck Surg* 1997;116:S1-S20.

Melen I: Chronic sinusitis: clinical and pathophysiological aspects. *Acta Otolaryngol Suppl (Stockh)* 1994;515:45-48.

Chapter 2

Anatomy, Physiology, and Pathophysiology

T he functions of the nose include olfaction, respiration, and defense. The functions of the four paired paranasal sinuses are not completely understood, but probably include regulation of intranasal pressure, olfaction, humidification and warming of inspired air, decreasing the weight of the skull to assist in head balance and flotation, shock absorption during head trauma, voice resonance, and secretion of mucus to keep the nasal passages moist (Table 1).

Anatomy

The four paired paranasal sinuses are the ethmoid, maxillary, frontal, and sphenoid sinuses (Figure 1). These are named after the cranial bones in which they are located. The sinuses normally contain air and are lined by ciliated, pseudostratified, columnar epithelium with interspersed goblet-type mucus-secreting cells.

Ethmoid Sinuses

The ethmoid sinuses begin their development during the third fetal month as evaginations of the lateral nasal wall. At birth, usually three or four ethmoid fluid cells are present. They are difficult to recognize on routine x-rays until an infant reaches 6 months of age. Only the ethmoid and the maxillary sinuses are significantly developed enough at birth to be clinically important. No significant growth of the sphenoid or frontal sinuses occurs until 3 years of age. The ethmoid si-

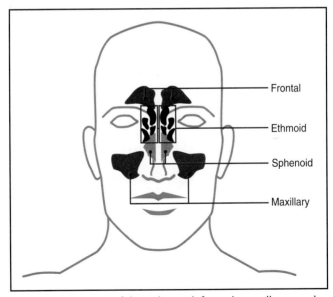

Figure 1: Depiction of the sphenoid, frontal, maxillary, and ethmoid sinuses.

nuses reach nearly adult size by age 12. They do not develop as single cavities, but rather as multiple cells, usually 10 to 15 on either side, that are separated by thin, bony septa.

The lateral wall of the ethmoid sinus is the lamina papyracea. This is a paper-thin bone that also forms the medial wall of the orbit. Superiorly, the roof of the ethmoid sinus is the fovea ethmoidalis, which is also the base of the skull. Medially along the roof of the ethmoid sinus is the thinner bone of the cribriform plate, which tends to lie 2 to 3 mm lower than the fovea ethmoidalis.

Two groups of cells exist within the ethmoid sinuses. The anterior group drains into the middle meatus and the posterior group drains into the superior meatus. The anterior and posterior ethmoid cells are divided by a plate of bone called the basal lamella (ground lamella). The anterior ethmoid cells can be further subdivided into frontal recess cells, infundibular cells, agger nasi cells, bullar cells, and conchal cells. The frontal recess is the most anterior and superior portion within the anterior ethmoid compartment, which communicates with the frontal sinus. The ethmoid infundibulum represents a cleft or space that is bounded medially by the uncinate process, laterally by the lamina papyracea, posteriorly by the ethmoid bulla, and opens into the middle meatus through the hiatus semilunaris. Agger nasi refers to a mound that may persist immediately anterior and superior to the insertion of the middle turbinate, and may be evident when a cell becomes pneumatized in that area. The ethmoid bulla is the largest and most constant air cell of the anterior ethmoid complex. Concha bullosa refers to pneumatization of the middle turbinate.

Maxillary Sinuses

The maxillary sinuses are believed to be the first of the sinuses to begin fetal development. A groove between the future uncinate process and ethmoid bulla begins to give rise to the maxillary sinus about the 65th day of gestation. At birth, the maxillary sinus is pea-sized and fluid-filled, making interpretation of plain x-rays difficult. The maxillary sinus undergoes two rapid growth spurts, between birth and age 3 years and between ages 7 and 18. The sinus becomes adult size by adolescence.

The roof of the maxillary sinus forms the floor of the orbit, while the floor of the maxillary sinus is formed by the alveolar process of the maxilla. In newborns and in small children, the floor of the maxillary sinus is above the floor of the nasal cavity, while in adults, the floor of the maxillary sinus is usually 5 to 10 mm below the floor of the nasal cavity. The 1st and 2nd molars and 2nd bicuspid teeth often project through the floor of the maxillary sinus, covered by the thin mucous membrane within the sinus. Infection around these tooth roots may therefore cause inflammation of the sinus mucous membranes. Removal of these teeth can cause fistulae and predispose to sinusitis. The anterior wall of the maxillary sinus separates the sinus from the cheek skin, while the posterior wall separates the sinus from the infratemporal and pterygomaxillary fossae.

The main ostium of the maxillary sinus is located in the superior and anterior aspect of the medial wall. Through this ostium the maxillary antrum communicates with the infundibulum in the middle meatus. Accessory ostia are usually acquired from chronic sinus infections.

Frontal Sinuses

Although the frontal sinuses begin development during the fourth gestational month, they are not clinically perceptible at birth. The frontal sinuses are believed to develop from pits or furrows in the frontal recess that were rudimentary anterior ethmoid cells. The frontal sinuses can rarely be demonstrated on plain x-ray before 2 years of age, when they begin a gradual vertical invasion of the frontal bone. Frontal sinus growth is complete by age 20. Failure to develop one or both frontal sinuses occurs in approximately 5% of the population.

The frontal sinus has an anterior and posterior table. The anterior table separates the sinus from the periosteum and forehead skin. The anterior table is twice as thick as the posterior table. The posterior table separates the sinus from the anterior cranial fossa. The frontal sinus is usually divided by intersinus

Table 2: Development of the Paranasal Sinuses

Sinus	Begins development	Status at birth	Development complete
Ethmoid	3rd month gestation	present	12 years
Maxillary	2nd month gestation	present	12 years
Frontal	4th month gestation	not present	20 years
Sphenoid	3rd month gestation	not present	15 years

septa and is rarely symmetric. The frontal sinus drains into the middle meatus via the frontal recess. The frontal recess opens either into the infundibulum or directly into the middle meatus.

Sphenoid Sinus

The sphenoid sinus begins development during the third gestational month as paired evaginations of mucosa in the posterior superior aspect of the nasal cavity, known as the sphenoethmoid recess. At birth, however, the sphenoid sinus is not perceptible, and growth of these evaginations does not begin until 3 years of age. Pneumatization usually becomes rapid after 7 years, to its adult size by 12 to 15 years. The left and right sides of the sphenoid sinus are separated by an intersinus septum and are usually asymmetric. The sphenoid sinus drains into the nose via the sphenoid ostium to the sphenoethmoid recess. Several important structures are related to the sphenoid sinus, including the optic nerve and pituitary superiorly, and the pons posteriorly. The cavernous sinus, superior orbital fissure, and internal carotid artery lie external and lateral to the sphenoid sinus. In half the population the internal carotid artery forms an indentation in the lateral wall of

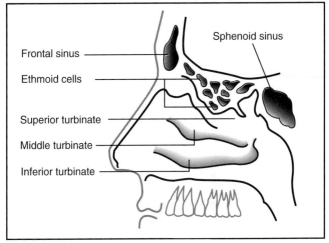

Figure 2: Side or parasagittal view of the sinuses and the turbinates.

the sphenoid sinus. Dehiscences may exist in the mucosa within the sphenoid and, therefore, much care must be taken when performing sphenoid surgery. Table 2 outlines development of the paranasal sinuses.

Lateral Nasal Wall and Ostiomeatal Complex (OMC)

The turbinates are projections from the lateral nasal wall (Figure 2). These are scrolls of bone, covered by a mucous membrane composed of ciliated, pseudostratified, columnar epithelium. The shape of the turbinates effectively increases the surface area of the mucous lining within the nose, allowing for greater filtration of particulate matter and greater efficiency in warming and humidifying inspired air. The inferior turbinate usually is the most prominent and obvious projection from the lateral wall of the nose on anterior rhinoscopy. There are usually three turbinates on each side of the nose: the inferior, middle, and superior. However, a small, fourth turbinate, the *supreme turbinate*, occasionally appears. *Agger nasi* refers to a small prominence often seen just anterior to the middle turbinate. This is an aeration in the bone or a "cell" that overlies the lacrimal sac. We believe agger nasi represents the remnant of another turbinate found in animals.

The meati are spaces created by the turbinates. The inferior meatus is the space between the inferior turbinate and the lateral nasal wall. The nasolacrimal duct drains into the inferior meatus at its anterior aspect. The middle meatus is the space between the middle turbinate and the lateral nasal wall. Likewise, the superior meatus is located between the superior turbinate and the lateral nasal wall.

The frontal, maxillary, and anterior ethmoid sinuses drain to a common channel (infundibulum) into the middle meatus. The drainage of these sinuses can be referred to as the *anterior sinus drainage system*. The borders of the infundibulum are the uncinate process anteriorly, the ethmoid bulla posteriorly, the lamina papyracea laterally, and the hiatus semilunaris medially. The uncinate process is a thin bone attached anteriorly to the lacrimal bone and inferiorly to the superior aspect of the inferior turbinate. The ethmoid bulla is the most anterior and most prominent ethmoid cell. The lamina papyracea is a paper-thin bone that separates the orbit from the ethmoid sinus. The hiatus semilunaris is the medial opening by which the secretions from the infundibulum are brought through the middle meatus into the nasal cavity.

The basal lamella, or ground lamella, is an important anatomic bony landmark that separates the anterior and posterior drainage systems. In the ethmoid sinus, the basal lamella separates the anterior ethmoid cavity from the posterior ethmoid cavity. The anterior ethmoid sinus drains into the middle meatus, while the posterior ethmoid sinus drains into the superior meatus. Finally, the sphenoid sinus drains posteriorly through the sphenoid ostium into the sphenoethmoid recess to the posterior nasal cavity.

The OMC is the key anatomic area addressed by endoscopic sinus surgeons. The OMC is bounded medially by the middle turbinate, posteriorly and superiorly by the basal lamella, and laterally by the lamina papyracea. Inferiorly and anteriorly, the OMC is open. This anatomic region therefore includes the anterior ethmoid sinus, ethmoid bulla, frontal recess, uncinate process, infundibulum, hiatus semilunaris, and middle meatus. Most authorities concur that disease or blockage of the OMC prevents effective mucociliary clearance, thus leading to bacterial sinusitis.

Physiology of the Paranasal Sinuses

The paranasal sinuses are lined with ciliated, pseudostratified, columnar epithelial cells (Figure 3). This respiratory-type epithelium is continuous with, and histologically similar to, that of the nasal cavity. The sinus mucosa contains interspersed, goblet-type mucus-secreting cells. These cells produce a biphasic blanket of mucus that serves to purify, humidify, and warm inspired air.

The normal physiology of the paranasal sinuses depends on three essential components: (1) normal sinus secretions; (2) functioning cilia; and (3) patent sinus ostia. These components allow for the continuous clearance of secretions (Table 3). The sinus mucosa secretes mucus into the sinus cavities. The mucus is propelled by ciliary action through natural ostia into the nasal cavity and nasopharynx. Conditions that interfere with any of the three components may predispose a patient to sinusitis.

The mucus blanket and ciliated epithelium constitute the mucociliary system. The mucus blanket is made up of two layers: a viscid superficial gel layer and a serous sol layer. The viscid layer traps particles such as bacteria and debris. The serous layer bathes the body of the cilia, allowing for efficient ciliary beat. The cilia have a quick, forward stroke and a slower recovery stroke in the opposite direction (Figure 4). During the forward stroke, the tips of the cilia contact the viscid layer, transporting it toward the ostia to remove particulate matter into the nasal cavity and nasopharynx. The cilia beat at a frequency of 1,000 strokes per minute, and the average mucociliary clearance time from an adult nose is about 10 minutes. The mucus blanket also contains lysozymes, secretory IgA and IgG, interferon, lactoferrin, and other enzymes to aid in defense.

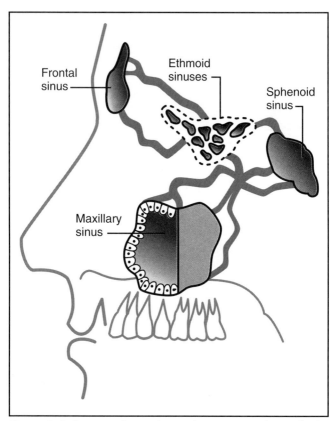

Figure 3: Side view of sinus lining showing pseudostratified columnar cells. Primary drainage problems of the ethmoid sinuses can cause secondary inflammation of the frontal, sphenoid, and maxillary sinuses.

Finally, for the mucociliary system to clear the secretions from the sinuses, there must be patent natural sinus ostia. This leads to the involvement of the OMC. The mucociliary transport from the frontal, maxillary, and anterior ethmoid sinuses converges in the OMC. It consists of the infundibulum, hiatus semilunaris, frontal recess, uncinate process, anterior ethmoid bulla, and the anterior wall of the middle turbinate. Our knowledge of the function of the OMC has markedly increased our understanding of sinus disease and how to treat it.

Studies by Messerklinger elucidated this process. He found that mucociliary clearance of the sinuses was disrupted when two mucosal surfaces came in contact. These areas are most likely to be at the narrow, mucosal-lined ostial channels

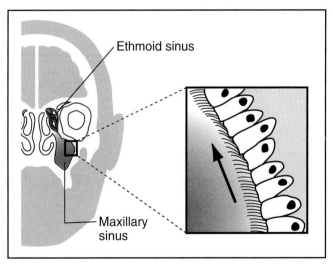

Figure 4: Ethmoid and maxillary sinuses, with inset depicting the surface cilia and how their constant beating motion (arrow) moves mucus from the sinuses to the nasal cavity.

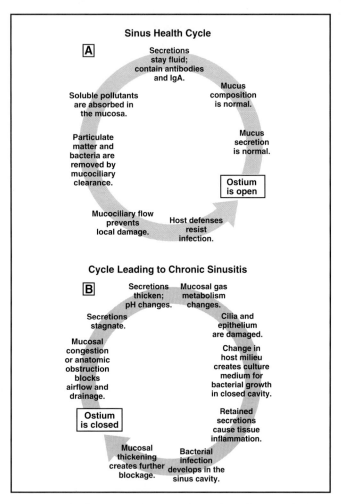

Figure 5: (A) Clearance of sinuses depends on functional cilia and mucous membranes and requires normal mucus production to maintain ostiomeatal patency. (B) Cycle of events that leads to chronic sinusitis begins with ostial blockage. Adapted from Kennedy DW, ed. *Sinus Disease: Guide to First-Line Management.* Darien, CT, Health Communications, 1994.

of the middle meatus. Any process that causes mucosal inflammation in the anterior ethmoid sinuses can occlude the other sinuses that drain at the OMC. We now know that severe mucosal disease of the maxillary and frontal sinuses can be resolved by controlling anterior ethmoid disease and achieving patency of the OMC. This allows for restoration of normal sinus aeration and mucociliary clearance.

Pathophysiology

The key factor in sinus disease is obstruction of the OMC. Many etiologic factors may contribute to OMC obstruction. In general, the OMC can be blocked by mucosal congestion or anatomic obstruction. The causes may be reversible with appropriate medical and surgical management. When obstruction occurs, the mucus is retained in the sinus cavity. These stagnant secretions thicken and provide a medium for bacterial growth. Obstruction also impairs aeration, or gas exchange within the sinus cavity. Absorption of trapped oxygen leads to hypoxia, which exacerbates sinus infection from both aerobic and anaerobic bacteria. These changes lead to damage and dysfunction of the cilia and epithelium. The retained secretions and infection lead to further tissue inflammation, which in turn leads to further ostial blockage. These events demonstrate a vicious circle that leads to chronic sinusitis. (Figure 5). Furthermore, any process that harms the mucociliary system (eg, cystic fibrosis, immotile cilia syndrome/Kartagener's syndrome) can result in the same cycle of events, leading to chronic sinusitis.

Selected Readings

Amedee RG: Sinus anatomy and function. In: Bailey BJ, ed. *Head and Neck Surgery—Otolaryngology*. Philadelphia, JB Lippincott, 1993, pp 342-349.

Facer GW, Kern EB: Sinusitis: current concepts and management. In: Bailey BJ, ed. *Head and Neck Surgery—Otolaryngology*. Philadelphia, JB Lippincott, 1993, pp 366-376.

Levine HL, May M, et al: Complex anatomy of the lateral nasal wall: simplified for the endoscopic sinus surgeon. In: Levine HL, May M, eds: *Endoscopic Sinus Surgery*. New York, Thieme Medical Publishers, 1993, pp 1-28.

Gwaltney JM Jr, Jones JG, Kennedy DW: Medical management of sinusitis: educational goals and management guidelines. The International Conference on Sinus Disease. *Ann Otol Rhinol Laryngol Suppl* 1995;167:22-30.

Kaliner MA, Osguthorpe JD, Fireman P, et al: Sinusitis: bench to bedside. Current findings, future directions. *Otolaryngol Head Neck Surg* 1997;116:S1-S20.

Knops JL, McCaffrey TV, Kern EB: Inflammatory diseases of the sinuses: physiology. Clinical applications. *Otolaryngol Clin North Am* 1993;26:517-534.

Shechtman FG, Kraus WM, Schaefer SD: Inflammatory diseases of the sinuses: anatomy. *Otolaryngol Clin North Am* 1993;26:509-516.

Stammberger HR, Kennedy DW: Paranasal sinuses: anatomic terminology and nomenclature. The Anatomic Terminology Group. *Ann Otol Rhinol Laryngol Suppl* 1995;167:7-16.

Chapter 3

Etiology

Rhinitis rarely exists without some degree of concomitant sinusitis, and vice versa, regardless of whether a virus, allergen, or nonallergic pollutant is the initial cause of inflammation. Mucociliary dysfunction or acquired IgG subtype deficiency may allow for the persistent growth of trapped bacteria within a sinus, leading to sinusitis. However, bacterial sinusitis most often follows obstruction of the ostiomeatal complex (OMC) from mucosal swelling. In addition, anatomic abnormalities such as polyps, tumors, foreign bodies, deviated nasal septum, and concha bullosae may cause obstruction with the same result. It is not unusual to see more than one contributing factor. Vasomotor rhinitis and iatrogenic factors (intranasal cocaine, rhinitis medicamentosa) are also potentially important, as are hormonal mucosal reactions associated with puberty, birth control pills, and senile rhinorrhea.

Researchers have recognized that secretory IgA deficiency can be important to patients with bacterial sinusitis, especially acute exacerbations of chronic sinusitis. Actually, IgA deficiency is always associated with an IgG subtype deficiency, which may be reversed by the monthly administration of intravenous immunoglobulin. This problem is more likely to be found in elderly patients who have failed to respond to adequate medical and surgical management. An infectious diseases specialist should be consulted for these patients.

Most anatomic abnormalities are easy to recognize and correct surgically. The common cold allergens and nonallergic pollutants are significant triggers and are not so easily controlled. Also, there is no vaccine against rhinoviruses. House dust and dust mites will never be totally eliminated, and irritants such as cigarette smoke, perfume, toxic chemicals, and other pollutants remain a problem for many patients.

Most episodes of acute sinusitis follow the common cold. The resident or colonizing microorganisms (mainly bacteria) in the nose and sinus mucosa would be expected to cause most episodes of sinusitis, but the role of viruses in primary infection has not been well studied. However, sinus aspirates from some patients with acute sinusitis have grown influenza, parainfluenza, and rhinoviruses. Magnetic resonance imaging (MRI) and computed tomography (CT) of the sinuses in patients with the common cold from rhinoviruses typically are abnormal, showing mucosal thickening and fluid accumulation, essentially the same as in bacterial sinusitis. It is well known that viral infections tend to destroy the cilia of the mucous membranes, and approximately 6 weeks are required for regeneration. Many clinicians believe that this is a predisposing factor for a bacterial sinusitis superinfection in patients who have mucus flow obstruction.

The sinuses produce 1 to 2 L of mucus per day, most of which is swallowed without awareness. Nasal mucus has a bacterial concentration of 10,000 to 100,000 bacteria/mL. Five times more strict anaerobes than aerobes and facultative anaerobes appear in this mucus, which is not surprising considering that mucosal surfaces are involved. The anterior nares are most commonly colonized with *Staphylococcus aureus*, but Enterobacteriaceae are also found, especially in patients who are immunocompromised (eg, diabetes mellitus, hemodialysis, AIDS, nursing home residents recently discharged from the hospital).

The microbiology of sinusitis remains an area of some disagreement. In general, infectious disease workers have required sinus puncture and aspiration for quantitative culture to confirm microbiologic etiology. Most studies have been

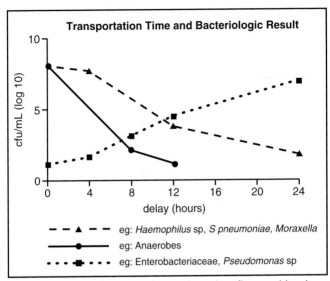

Figure 1: Bacteriologic results are heavily influenced by the duration of transportation of the specimen.

done on maxillary sinus secretions because of their accessibility. Even so, patients frequently resist this procedure. In expert hands, rigid endoscopy with culture of the OMC in acute maxillary sinusitis yields a sensitivity and specificity of 80% and 85% respectively, when compared with material aspirated from a sinus puncture for *Haemophilus influenzae*, *Streptococcus pneumoniae*, and *Moraxella catarrhalis*. Very few studies have been done looking for atypical organisms (*Mycoplasma pneumoniae*, *Chlamydia pneumoniae*, and *Legionella* species), but any infectious agent that produces disease in one part of the respiratory tract has the capability of producing disease in another part. Antimicrobial therapy for sinusitis has been largely empiric and based on relatively little data. The microbiologic etiology of most clinical acute sinusitis and acute exacerbations of sinusitis in patients with chronic sinusitis is never determined. Handling of the specimen also influences bacteriologic result (Figure 1).

Because of the number of antimicrobials used for sinusitis, coupled with increasing antimicrobial resistances, the pharmaceutical industry has remained active in looking for new agents to market for the disease. The FDA requires sinus puncture/aspiration to be done on a number of patients before a drug can be approved. As of November 1997, the FDA had approved a number of antimicrobials for use in acute sinusitis. They are amoxicillin/clavulanate (Augmentin®), levofloxacin (Levaquin®), loracarbef (Lorabid®), clarithromycin (Biaxin®), cefprozil (Cefzil®), cefuroxime axetil (Ceftin®), and ciprofloxacin (Cipro®). None has been approved for chronic sinusitis.

Three pharmaceutical companies have recently pursued FDA approval for an antimicrobial for sinusitis therapy. This has resulted in a large body of microbiologic data, much of which has not been published. Nevertheless, review of data from several thousand patients confirms the earlier studies showing the importance of *H influenzae*, *S pneumoniae*, *M catarrhalis*, and *S aureus* as the chief bacterial pathogens isolated by culture from patients with acute sinusitis or acute exacerbations in patients with chronic sinusitis. Anaerobic bacteria are more commonly cultured in patients with chronic sinusitis, but were not a significant factor in patients with acute exacerbations of underlying chronic sinusitis. Unfortunately, the roles of *M pneumoniae*, *C pneumoniae*, and *Legionella* species, if any, have yet to be defined.

A problem in deciding the relative importance of any of the four main bacterial pathogens is that although *S pneumoniae* appears to show no seasonal variation, *H influenzae* in one study was more prevalent in the late winter than in early spring. In addition, there may be geographic variations and, obviously, underlying diseases are critical. For example, acute sinusitis in the hemodialysis patient should increase the concern that *S aureus* might be playing a role.

We might assume that nasal carriage of a bacterial pathogen that subsequently causes acute sinusitis is the reason that those persons have those organisms, whereas a noncarrier would not. However, no data are available to support this assumption. These data are difficult to acquire because the patient may be carrying few organisms, thus escaping surveillance culturing.

A recent study from Finland comparing the nasal bacterial flora in healthy subjects with that of patients with acute maxillary sinusitis found that the nasal culture grew the same pathogen as that found in a sinus aspirate culture 91% of the time. The predictive value of a pathogen-positive nasal culture was 95% for *S pyogenes,* followed by 78% for *H influenzae* and 69% *for S pneumoniae*. It was only 20% for *M catarrhalis*. *S pyogenes* is not a major sinus pathogen in the United States.

Because of their inconvenience and cost, routine smears and cultures will unlikely be performed for patients with suspected community-acquired sinusitis or acute exacerbations of chronic sinusitis.

Studies of the microbiology of chronic sinusitis have established a role for anaerobic bacteria. The anaerobic microorganisms most commonly found are the same found less frequently in acute sinusitis, including anaerobic streptococci, *Bacteroides* species, and *Fusobacterium*. In a carefully performed study in 1974 by Frederich and Braude, cultures were obtained from 83 patients with chronic sinusitis. The cultures were taken in the operating room under sterile conditions from the patients' infected sinuses. Twenty-four (29%) had only anaerobic bacteria cultured, including *Corynebacterium*, *Bacteroides* species, and anaerobic streptococci. Other studies involving chronic sinusitis found up to 40% with no growth. Because of the fastidious nature of anaerobic bacteria, it is possible that these bacteria were present but not identified. With chronic sinusitis, it is not unusual for more than one bacterium to be isolated. Whether or not this is a factor in pathogenesis is difficult to determine, but obviously has implications for antimicrobial therapy.

Potential fungal pathogens, especially molds such as *Phycomycetes* (*Mucor*, *Rhizopus*, etc) and *Aspergillus* species, are commonly inhaled and may reach the sinuses. Disease production is unlikely unless the patient is immunocompromised. Fungal infections are certainly a risk for patients with uncontrolled diabetes mellitus or AIDS, those on prolonged immunosuppression therapy (especially transplant recipients), and those on prolonged courses of broad-spectrum antibiotics for respiratory tract infection prevention (cystic fibrosis, etc). Interestingly, despite the common occurrence of oral candidiasis, *Candida* species and other yeasts are not commonly associated with sinusitis. Allergic fungal sinusitis from *Aspergillus* species is similar to allergic bronchopulmonary aspergillosis, with the secretions containing eosinophils, Charcot-Leyden crystals, and fungal hyphae. Antifungal therapy with itraconazole (Sporanox®) is being evaluated for allergic bronchopulmonary aspergillosis. Tissue invasion does not occur in either condition.

The recognized microbial etiology of sinusitis consists of rhinoviruses, bacteria, and fungi. Other microorganisms such as *C pneumoniae* and *M pneumoniae* are likely to be important as well. Of the bacteria involved, it appears that *H influenzae* and *S pneumoniae* are the most important pathogens in acute sinusitis. *M catarrhalis* and *S aureus* play a variable role. In addition, anaerobes and other gram-negative bacilli may be important in chronic sinusitis. Because of the emergence of microbial resistance to available agents for the treatment of sinusitis (beta-lactamase-producing bacteria, penicillin-resistant *S pneumoniae*, methicillin-resistant *S aureus*, and others), the development of new agents should increase our understanding of the microbiology of sinusitis.

Selected Readings

Gwaltney JM Jr: Acute community-acquired sinusitis. *Clin Infect Dis* 1996;23:1209-1225.

Donald TJ, Gluckman JL, Rice DH: *The Sinuses.* New York, Raven Press, 1995.

Chapter 4

Classification

Sinusitis may be chronologically classified into 5 categories: (1) acute; (2) recurrent acute; (3) subacute; (4) chronic; and (5) acute exacerbation of chronic (Table 1). *Acute* sinusitis is sudden in onset and its signs and symptoms may last up to 4 weeks. The diagnosis of *recurrent acute* sinusitis is made when 4 or more episodes of acute sinusitis occur in one year, without intervening signs and symptoms of sinusitis while off antibiotics. *Subacute* sinusitis represents the gray area between acute and chronic sinusitis, and is present when the signs and symptoms last 4 to 12 weeks. *Chronic* sinusitis is found when the signs and symptoms are present for more than 12 weeks. *Acute exacerbation of chronic* sinusitis represents sudden worsening of chronic sinusitis with return to baseline chronic signs and symptoms after treatment. Clinicians should be able to differentiate these categories because doing so provides the basis for determining the therapeutic approaches to each condition. For example, uncomplicated acute sinusitis usually responds to adequate medical treatment, whereas surgical treatment must be considered in complicated or recurrent acute and chronic sinusitis.

The diagnosis of sinusitis is made on the basis of the signs, symptoms, and findings. The signs and symptoms of sinusitis include major and minor ones. These vary slightly depending

Table 1: Classification of Sinusitis

Classification	Duration
Acute	10 days - 4 weeks or exacerbation of initial URI symptoms after 5 days
Recurrent acute	4 or more episodes of acute per year
Subacute	4 - 12 weeks
Chronic	>12 weeks
Acute exacerbation of chronic	sudden worsening, with return to baseline chronic sinusitis after treatment

on the source. Major criteria generally include facial pain/pressure, facial congestion/fullness, nasal congestion/obstruction, nasal discharge/purulence/discolored postnasal drainage, hyposmia/anosmia, fever (for acute sinusitis), and purulence on intranasal examination (Table 2). Minor criteria include headache, fever (for subacute and chronic sinusitis), halitosis, fatigue, dental pain, cough, and ear pain/pressure/fullness (Table 3). Criteria more specific to children include cough and irritability. A *strong* history consistent with a diagnosis of sinusitis is indicated by the presence of: (1) 2 major criteria or (2) 1 major and 2 minor criteria. A *suggestive* history is indicated by the presence of (1) 1 major criterion or (2) 2 minor criteria (Table 4).

Certain diagnostic measures can provide helpful confirmatory information. Nasal cytology showing abundant neutrophils and Waters' view by plain film showing mucosal thickening, air-fluid level, or opacification may aid in the diagnosis of acute sinusitis. However, the consensus among experts is that imaging studies are not universally necessary. The imaging modality of choice is the computed tomography (CT) scan, which is recommended primarily in evaluating the

Table 2: Major Criteria of Sinusitis

- Facial pain/pressure*
- Facial congestion/fullness
- Nasal congestion/obstruction
- Nasal discharge/purulence/ discolored postnasal drainage
- Hyposmia/anosmia
- Fever (for acute sinusitis)**
- Purulence on intranasal examination

* requires a second major criterion to constitute a suggestive history
** requires a second major criterion to constitute a strong history

extent and severity of disease in chronic sinusitis, recurrent acute sinusitis, and complicated sinusitis.

The diagnosis of acute sinusitis is made when the signs and symptoms persist longer than a typical viral upper respiratory tract infection (10 days to 4 weeks) or when the signs

Table 3: Minor Criteria of Sinusitis

- Headache
- Fever (for subacute and chronic)
- Halitosis
- Fatigue
- Dental pain
- Cough
- Ear pain/pressure/fullness

Table 4: Diagnosis of Sinusitis Based on Major and Minor Criteria

Strong history requires the presence of:
   2 major criteria or 1 major and 2 or more minor criteria

Suggestive history requires the presence of:
   1 major criterion or 2 or more minor criteria

and symptoms become exacerbated after the initial 5 days. Acute bacterial sinusitis usually follows a viral upper respiratory tract infection (URI). Typically, acute sinusitis resolves with medical therapy, resulting in no significant mucosal damage.

Four or more episodes of acute sinusitis per year constitute recurrent acute sinusitis. These episodes resolve with medical therapy, and are separated by symptom-free intervals while off antibiotics. Recurrent acute sinusitis requires further work-up to uncover anatomic or systemic underlying factors. Certainly, referral to an otolaryngologist is necessary.

After 4 weeks, acute sinusitis that has not resolved may be classified as subacute sinusitis. Subacute sinusitis is a rarely used term, but represents sinusitis that lasts 4 to 12 weeks. Subacute sinusitis may represent acute sinusitis that has either been inappropriately treated or not treated at all. Symptoms become less severe. For example, fever is not considered a major criteria for the diagnosis of subacute sinusitis. Generally, adequate medical treatment of subacute sinusitis should lead to complete resolution with no resultant mucosal damage.

Chronic sinusitis is most commonly defined as persistent signs and symptoms of sinusitis for more than 3 months, with or without a constant need for antibiotic therapy. Chronic sinusitis may be punctuated with acute exacerbations (accounting for the fifth classification). Chronic sinusitis requires evaluation by an otolaryngologist to aid in identifying etiologic factors and to determine the need for endoscopic sinus surgery. Surgery focuses on alleviation of ostial obstruction to permit aeration of the sinuses and regeneration of damaged mucosa.

Selected Readings

Dana ST: Out of committee. *Bull Am Acad Otolaryngol Head Neck Surg* 1994;13:12-14.

Lanza DC, Kennedy DW: Adult rhinosinusitis defined. *Otolaryngol Head Neck Surg* 1997;117:51-57.

Lund VJ, Kennedy DW: Quantification for staging sinusitis. *Ann Otol Rhinol Laryngol Suppl* 1995;167:17-21.

Shapiro GG, Rachelefsky GS: Introduction and definition of sinusitis. *J Allergy Clin Immunol* 1992;90:417-418.

Chapter 5

Diagnosis

Acute sinusitis and acute exacerbations of chronic sinusitis can have similar symptoms and physical findings. Most patients who present to their primary care physician for acute sinus problems have allergy, rhinoviruses, or bacteria as the cause. This chapter addresses acute bacterial sinusitis and chronic sinusitis.

Acute Sinusitis

History

The patient's history can reveal underlying causes of acute sinusitis. Factors that can lead to ostial obstruction include viral upper respiratory tract infection, allergic rhinitis, vasomotor rhinitis, barotrauma, and mucosal hypertrophy. Furthermore, mechanical obstruction can be caused by choanal atresia, nasal polyps, deviated nasal septum, a foreign body, trauma, and tumors. Recent dental work or infections can introduce bacteria into the maxillary sinus. Sinus colonization with bacteria not commonly found in the sinuses can occur with instrumentation such as nasogastric intubation in a septic patient, or in a patient with connective tissue disease or immunodeficiency, including AIDS. All of these factors should be kept in mind during history taking and during physical examination.

Primary care physicians can easily recognize the patient with acute bacterial sinusitis. Typically, the patient has an antecedent viral upper respiratory tract infection whose symptoms have failed to clear after numerous over-the-counter and home remedies. Patients with medical insurance usually will not allow these symptoms to persist longer than 2 or 3 weeks before seeking professional advice. Others wait up to 2 months and account for the classification of acute sinusitis for patients symptomatic less than 8 weeks. Community-acquired bacterial sinusitis is not unusual as a complication of maxillary dental sepsis or allergy. Patients with acute bacterial sinusitis complain of facial pain that is aggravated by bending over, a yellow-greenish nasal discharge, nasal obstruction, unpleasant breath and taste, increased postnasal mucus (especially in the upright position), headache, and cough. Many patients also complain of chills and fever.

Because purulent nasal discharge and facial pain are the most common clinical findings in acute bacterial sinus infection, the location of the facial pain may suggest which sinuses are involved. Pain in the cheeks suggests maxillary sinusitis, whereas pain in the forehead or medial orbit suggests frontal sinusitis. Medial canthus pain suggests ethmoid sinusitis, and retro-orbital or occipital pain is associated with sphenoid sinusitis.

It is not surprising that confusion exists about differentiation from the common cold, especially if the patient is seen within the first week of the onset of the cold. Rhinoviral infection produces a rhinosinusitis. Computed tomography studies in otherwise healthy adults with colds reveal thick nasal walls, engorged turbinates, and occluded maxillary ostia. Thick secretions are trapped in the maxillary sinuses (and others as well), creating an environment for bacterial growth and for producing sinus pressure. These symptoms usually resolve within a week if no bacterial sinusitis develops. Patients who develop bacterial sinusitis seek help because of fever, headache, facial pain, or nasal obstruction that interferes with sleep and that is not relieved by over-the-counter preparations.

Physical examination usually reveals low-grade fever in an obviously uncomfortable patient. Fever greater than 100° F occurs in only 50% of adult patients. Pressure over the involved sinuses is frequently painful, and purulent nasal discharge is readily apparent. A careful examination of the oral cavity is also required, looking for abnormal maxillary molars and posterior pharyngeal mucus. The tympanic membranes should also be examined for evidence of otitis media.

If a windowless room is available, transillumination of the maxillary and frontal sinuses may be useful. This is especially helpful if the two sides transilluminate differently, although a frontal sinus may not be developed, giving a false impression that it is filled with fluid. Imaging techniques are addressed in Chapter 6; however, it is unlikely in this era of managed care that any procedure would be done unless surgery is being considered, or the patient is immunocompromised or ill enough to consider hospitalization.

Signs and symptoms that require further diagnostic evaluation and consideration for hospitalization include recent discharge from the hospital where an intubation, feeding, or suction device was in the nasal cavity (nosocomial sinusitis possible); an immunocompromised patient (a solid organ transplant recipient is more likely to have *Aspergillus* sinusitis); a patient with severe headache or mental changes (meningitis possible); or severe facial pain suggesting frontal or sphenoid sinusitis, especially in a male adolescent.

In an attempt to aid primary care physicians in diagnosing sinusitis, a study by Williams and coworkers at a Veterans Administration Hospital walk-in clinic confirmed that male adult patients with sinus symptoms could be accurately stratified as having high, intermediate, or low probability of sinusitis based on clinical impression. The presence of maxillary toothache, history of poor response to nasal decongestants or antihistamines, colored nasal discharge reported by the patient, mucopurulent nasal discharge seen during the examination, and transillumination abnormalities were independent predictors of sinusitis. Therefore, the presence of all five was associated with high probability of sinusitis. Expansion of these studies to other populations (women, pediatrics, etc) and in different geographic areas would be interesting.

Table 1: Etiologic Factors in Sinusitis

Inflammatory Factors

Upper respiratory tract infection
Allergic rhinitis
Vasomotor rhinitis
Recent dental work
Barotrauma

Systemic Factors

Immunodeficiency
Immotile cilia syndrome
Kartagener's syndrome
Cystic fibrosis
Rhinitis secondary to pregnancy
Hypothyroidism

Mechanical Factors

Choanal atresia
Sinonasal polyps
Deviated nasal septum
Foreign body
Trauma
Tumor
Nasogastric tube
Turbinate hypertrophy
Concha bullosa
Adenoid hypertrophy

Medications

Rhinitis medicamentosa
• overuse of topical decongestants
Beta-blockers
Birth control pills
Antihypertensives
Aspirin intolerance
Cocaine abuse

Chronic Sinusitis

Chronic sinusitis is present when there are persistent signs and symptoms of sinusitis for 3 months or longer. The more physiologic definition of chronic sinusitis is disease in which the mucosal damage is no longer reversible despite appropriate medical therapy. Definitive cure will most likely require surgery that addresses at least the ostiomeatal complex (OMC). All patients with the diagnosis of chronic sinusitis or recurrent acute sinusitis should be evaluated by an otolaryngologist. The approach they use is summarized in this chapter.

History

Patient history is critically important. By history alone, a clinician can determine the presence of significant symptoms of sinusitis, such as nasal congestion or obstruction, nasal discharge (including color and quality of secretions), facial pains, pressure, headaches, olfactory disturbance, fever, halitosis, postnasal drip, sore throat, and cough. The history, combined with the physical examination, may provide enough information to suspect sinusitis and begin medical therapy. Most authors consider nasal congestion/obstruction, facial pain/pressure, facial congestion/pressure, nasal discharge/purulence/discolored postnasal drainage, and hyposmia/anosmia important major criteria associated with a clinical diagnosis of sinusitis. Minor criteria include headache, halitosis, fatigue, dental pain, cough, and ear pain/pressure/fullness. Fever is a major criterion for acute sinusitis and is a minor criterion for chronic sinusitis. The presence of two major criteria or one major plus two or more minor criteria indicate a *strong* history for sinusitis. One major criterion or two or more minor criteria indicate a *suggestive* history for sinusitis. Diagnostic tests can provide confirmatory information. Chronic sinusitis is determined either by the duration of the problem or by failure of medical therapy to eradicate disease (signs and symptoms present <12 weeks). Patients with chronic sinusitis generally present with mucopurulent discharge and mild nasal congestion, while systemic symptoms and pain are often absent.

The history often suggests the underlying causes of sinusitis (Table 1). Factors that can lead to ostial obstruction include viral upper respiratory tract infection, allergic rhinitis, vasomotor rhinitis, barotrauma, and mucosal hypertrophy. Furthermore, mechanical obstruction can be caused by choanal atresia, nasal polyps, deviated septum, foreign body, trauma, and tumors. Recent dental work or infections can introduce bacteria into the maxillary sinus. Sinus colonization with abnormal bacteria may also occur in a patient who has a nasogastric tube, in a septic patient, or in one with collagen vascular disease or immunodeficiency, including AIDS. Recurrent and chronic sinusitis may be caused by defects in mucociliary clearance such as in cystic fibrosis, Kartagener's syndrome, IgA deficiencies, and ciliary dysmotility. All of the above factors should be kept in mind during history taking and physical examination.

Physical Findings

The diagnosis of chronic sinusitis is determined by a careful history and physical examination, and confirmed by testing such as culture and imaging. Because complications of chronic sinusitis may include orbital, intracranial, and systemic complications, it is important to completely assess the patient, noting his or her general health and condition and general mental status. A complete head and neck examination should always be performed, including examination of the orbits, extraocular motility, pupillary response, vision, and cranial nerve function. The location of tenderness or pressure should be noted with palpation/percussion over the frontal sinuses, cheeks (maxillary sinuses), and medial orbit (ethmoid sinuses). Periorbital swelling or erythema can occur in the child with ethmoid sinusitis. Malodorous breath also commonly occurs in children. The ear examination is important because otitis media can occur with sinusitis. In a complete examination, the nasopharynx should be assessed for postnasal drainage and for obstruction by adenoid hypertrophy, tumor, or choanal atresia.

The nasal examination should include anterior rhinoscopy with good lighting. A topical decongestant, such as oxymetazoline or phenylephrine, is useful because it can shrink the mucosa and allow better visualization. The clinician should note whether the mucosa demonstrates a vasoconstrictive response to the topical decongestant. This helps determine whether nasal obstruction is caused by mucosal reaction or is strictly structural. The condition of the mucosal linings should be inspected, noting any edema, erythema, or purulent secretion. Inflammation of the mucosa may result from inhaled irritants, infected secretions, or response to allergens. Chronic inflammation may lead to the formation of polypoid mucosa or polyps. When ciliary activity is diminished, the nasal secretions may appear dry. Dry secretions may also be seen as a response to cold or hot air through the nasal passages. When purulent secretions become dehydrated, they can manifest as crusts. The location of pus within the nasal cavity may indicate which sinuses are involved. Pus may be seen in the middle meatus with infection of the frontal, maxillary, or anterior ethmoid sinuses. Purulent secretions located high along the lateral nasal wall, coming from the superior meatus, would be consistent with infection in the posterior ethmoid sinuses. Sphenoid sinusitis would be evident from pus at the sphenoethmoid recess in the posterior aspect of the nasal cavity. Of course, if the ostia are severely blocked, pus will be retained within the affected sinus cavity and may not readily be seen on examination. Furthermore, these precise locations are not easily delineated by anterior rhinoscopy, but greater diagnostic accuracy can be achieved with nasal endoscopy. Obviously, with the constraints of training and time, most primary care physicians would be unlikely to perform the extensive nasal examination as outlined. We strongly recommend early referral of patients with chronic sinusitis to an otolaryngologist.

Nasal Endoscopy

Nasal endoscopy allows for more detailed examination of the nasal cavities and can be performed with a flexible fiberoptic or rigid endoscope. The flexible fiberoptic endoscope is useful in examining the superior aspects of the nasal cavity and the nasopharynx and in evaluating postnasal drip because its flexibility allows examination of the structures all the way down to the vocal cords. The rigid endoscopes are now advocated for diagnostic purposes by most otolaryngologists who are experienced with functional endoscopic sinus surgery (FESS). The rigid endoscopes provide greater definition than the flexible scopes. The rigid scopes come with 0-degree, 30-degree, or 70-degree fixed-angle lenses. Topical decongestant and topical anesthesia are applied. Spraying the nose with 1% phenylephrine and 2% tetracaine (Pontocaine®) often is sufficient to make the patient comfortable for a complete office examination with nasal endoscopy. If necessary, additional comfort can be effectively achieved by placing 4% topical lidocaine (Xylocaine®) on a cotton pledget into the nasal cavity for 5 minutes.

After appropriate decongestant and topical anesthesia, the 4-mm nasal endoscope with 0-degree or 30-degree lens is passed into the nasal cavity. Examination of the inferior, middle, and superior turbinates; septum; posterior choanae; nasopharynx; sphenoethmoid recess; frontal recess; uncinate process; hiatus semilunaris; ethmoid bulla; and accessory ostia is possible with marked accuracy and detail. The quality of the mucosa and secretions are noted. The septum is evaluated for deviations, which not only can cause nasal obstruction, but also can impede the middle turbinate and lead to narrowing of the middle meatus and the OMC. The middle turbinate is evaluated to see whether its shape and size have caused narrowing of the middle meatus. A paradoxical middle turbinate can cause narrowing because its convex side protrudes into the lateral nasal wall. A large middle turbinate can cause nasal and OMC obstruction. A large middle turbinate may represent a concha bullosa, which is an aerated middle turbinate. The middle meatus is evaluated for the presence of narrowing, mucosal swelling, polyps or polypoid degeneration, and purulent secretions. Within the middle meatus, the uncinate process and the ethmoid bulla may be evaluated. More superiorly, the superior turbinate may be seen. Purulent secretions in the superior meatus may represent drainage from the posterior ethmoid or sphenoethmoid recess (from the sphenoid sinus). The inferior turbinate can be followed all the way back to the choana; the otolaryngologist should carefully note whether it causes obstruction of the nasal cavity. In the posterior nasal cavity, the sphenoethmoid recess and choana can be evaluated. Finally, the nasopharynx and the torus tubarius are evaluated for lesions or inflammation. Inflammation of the torus tubarius can lead to eustachian tube obstruction and cause middle ear manifestations.

Sinus Puncture

In most cases, the diagnosis of chronic sinusitis is made by the history and physical examination only. Sinus puncture is occasionally used to obtain material for bacteriologic studies in either acute or chronic sinusitis. This is performed by first providing local anesthesia to the lateral nasal wall in the inferior meatus. Next, a needle or trocar is inserted at the anterior aspect of the inferior meatus through the lateral nasal wall into the maxillary sinus. Purulent secretion may be aspirated for culture. Saline may be passed through the trocar to irrigate the sinus and flush secretions through the natural ostium into the nasal cavity. These procedures are generally reserved for refractory cases.

Transillumination

Transillumination is a diagnostic method in which a flashlight is placed over the suspected maxillary sinus (over the cheek) and checked for dullness of the light transmission. This test is based on the idea that a fluid-filled sinus will not transmit as much light as an empty sinus. Some clinicians like to use transillumination for evaluation of the frontal sinus by placing the light against the medial floor. This test is rarely used because the findings from transillumination do not necessarily accurately correlate with actual findings. However, some clinicians still find it useful in determining the resolution of sinusitis during treatment.

Mucociliary Clearance

The saccharin time test can determine abnormal mucociliary clearance. A drop of liquid saccharin placed on the inferior turbinate should elicit a distinctive taste within 12 minutes. Abnormal test results may be seen in smokers and others with altered ciliary function, and particularly in patients with recent upper respiratory infection. An abnormal result should alert the examiner to search for processes that may alter secretion clearance. An inferior or middle turbinate biopsy placed in glutaraldehyde can be examined by electron microscopy for the presence of abnormal cilia, as seen in ciliary dyskinesia or immotile cilia syndrome. History of infertility, abnormal sperm motility, and chest x-ray demonstrating situs inversus indicate possible ciliary abnormalities. Immunodeficient patients may demonstrate altered clearance. In cystic fibrosis, mucociliary clearance is impaired because of increased viscosity of the secretions.

Laboratory Testing

Several laboratory tests should be considered in the work-up of patients with chronic sinusitis or recurrent acute sinusitis. These include serum immunoglobulin levels, erythrocyte sedimentation rate (ESR), complete blood count (CBC), and sweat chloride. Serum immunoglobulin levels, including IgG subclasses, may reveal an underlying deficiency. IgA deficiency is found in 0.2% of Caucasians and, therefore, is occasionally seen as a complicating factor in chronic sinusitis. Levels of IgG1 in deficient patients may be augmented by immunization with diphtheria toxoid conjugate (ProHIBiT® *Haemophilus influenzae* type b conjugate vaccine), an IgG1 antigen. Furthermore, these immunizations provide patients with antibodies to *H influenzae* and *Streptococcus pneumoniae*, which are the most common pathogens in sinusitis. Immunoglobulin deficiency should be managed by the allergist/immunologist or infectious disease specialist. An elevated ESR may indicate a systemic disease such as Wegener's granulomatosis. When HIV infection is suspected, an HIV antibody test should be performed. Sweat chloride testing is performed to rule out cystic fibrosis, especially in children with nasal polyps or chronic or recurrent sinusitis.

Allergy Testing

During history taking, underlying allergies may be suspected in the patient who describes itchy or watery eyes, itchy nose, frequent sneezing, rhinorrhea with nasal congestion, or itchy palate. Patients suspected of having underlying allergies should be considered for evaluation by an allergist. These patients are treated with topical nasal corticosteroid spray or cromolyn spray (Nasalcrom®) and oral, nonsedating antihistamines; when these treatments fail, patients should undergo allergy testing. Oral antihistamines are specifically reserved for sinusitis patients *with underlying allergies*, because the drying effect of antihistamines may thicken secretions and can be otherwise detrimental in treating sinusitis. Patients with seasonal allergies should avoid pollens. Patients with perennial allergies should avoid exposure to dust, mold, and pet dander. Appropriate environmental avoidance measures should be followed based on radioallergosorbent test (RAST) or skin testing. Immunotherapy is used in patients with severe allergies or allergies that do not improve with medical therapy or avoidance measures.

Radiography

Plain sinus x-rays are still probably the most common (but not the most appropriate) imaging studies for evaluation of sinus disease. The standard plain radiograph sinus series includes: (1) Caldwell (anteroposterior); (2) Waters'; (3) submentovertex; and (4) lateral images. The Caldwell and Waters' views demonstrate the frontal and maxillary sinuses. Ethmoid sinuses are poorly visualized because of superimposition. The lateral and submentovertex views are useful for viewing the sphenoid sinus. Plain x-rays may help evaluate the patient suspected of having acute sinusitis, although this diagnosis is usually simply made based on history and physical findings. Furthermore, plain x-rays have limited value for the evaluation of chronic sinusitis. Plain x-rays provide poor visualization of the OMC, which is the key region in sinusitis. CT scan has replaced x-rays as the imaging study of choice for chronic sinusitis. While nasal endoscopy is valuable in imaging surface anatomy, CT scan (coronal views of the paranasal sinuses) can image the underlying sinus anatomy in detail, including the entire OMC. The combination of nasal endoscopy and CT scan in the evaluation of chronic sinus disease allows for precise diagnosis and treatment. Imaging studies are addressed in further detail in the next chapter.

Suggested Readings

Current perspectives on the management of chronic sinusitis: proceedings of a roundtable, October 16, 1994. Scienta Healthcare Education, 1995.

Facer GW, Kern EB: Sinusitis: current concepts and management. In: Bailey BJ, ed. *Head and Neck Surgery—Otolaryngology*. Philadelphia, JB Lippincott, 1993, pp 366-376.

Lanza DC, Kennedy DW: Adult rhinosinusitis defined. *Otolaryngol Head Neck Surg* 1997;117:S1-S7.

Gwaltney JM Jr, Jones JG, Kennedy DW: Medical management of sinusitis: educational goals and management guidelines. The International Conference on Sinus Disease. *Ann Otol Rhinol Laryngol Suppl* 1995;167:22-30.

May M, Mester SJ, Levine HL: Office evaluation of nasosinus disorders: patient selection for endoscopic sinus surgery. In: Levine HL, May M, eds: *Endoscopic Sinus Surgery*. New York, Thieme Medical Publishers, 1993, pp 60-90.

Shapiro GG, Rachelefsky GS: Introduction and definition of sinusitis. *J Allergy Clin Immunol* 1992;90:417-418.

Chapter 6

Imaging of the Sinuses

The paranasal sinuses are pneumatized bony structures that surround the nasal vault. They consist of two frontal, two maxillary, one sphenoid, and two ethmoid components. The ethmoid sinuses contain multiple air cells and are divided into anterior and posterior segments. The paranasal sinuses may have evolved as protection for the brain by providing an air-filled crushable barrier to absorb the energy from an assault. The reflex to turn and visualize an oncoming threat dictates the placement of this shock absorber: anteriorly, within the facial bones; surrounding the orbits; and in front of the brain. The paranasal sinuses' ability to dissipate great force is akin to the designs of modern automobiles that have crushable front and back ends that protect the contents of the passenger compartment. The paranasal sinuses also play several physiologic roles. These include humidifying, warming, and removing particulate matter from the air. Humidification and warming are accomplished by the watery secretions of serous glands. These serous glands can produce 1 to 2 L of secretions per day. The secretions of the goblet cells and mucous glands facilitate the removal of particulate matter. This mucus is very effective, trapping up to 80% of particles larger than 3 to 5 microns. This includes not only inorganic pathogens, but also up to 75% of the bacteria entering the nose. This mucous blanket is a very dynamic structure,

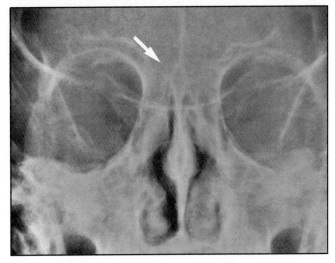

Figure 1: Plain radiograph in a patient with cystic fibrosis. Modified Caldwell's view demonstrating aplastic frontal sinuses (white arrow).

continuously renewing itself every 10 to 20 minutes. The mucous blanket also defends the body against infection. Besides trapping organic pathogens, the blanket constitutes a rich immunologic investment within the sinus mucosa. When exposed to the trapped antigens, it can further prepare a defense by stimulating the immunologic system. The ciliated epithelium continuously beats, propelling the mucus in a synchronized fashion toward the ostium of each sinus. These ostia drain into the nasal vault. The mucus then is propelled to the nasopharynx, to be swallowed into the digestive tract. At this point, the acidic secretions from the stomach can help destroy the inhaled pathogens. Other hypothetical functions of the paranasal sinuses, such as enhancement of vocal tone or depth, have no scientific basis.

The paranasal sinuses are not all present at birth. Rather, they develop in a predictable fashion. In the newborn, there is rudimentary pneumatization of both the maxillary and eth-

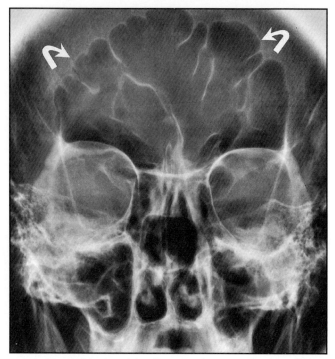

Figure 2: Modified Caldwell's view demonstrating extensive pneumatization of the frontal sinuses (curved white arrows). Sinus pneumatization varies greatly, and this finding is of no particular significance.

moid sinuses, with subsequent pneumatization of the sphenoid and frontal sinuses at approximately 3 and 6 years of age. Both the timing and extent of sinus development can undergo normal variations. Sinuses may normally be hypoplastic or aplastic. This variable degree of pneumatization or development is most commonly seen in the frontal sinuses. However, poorly pneumatized sinuses may also indicate an underlying disease process in which mucus production or clearance is altered (Figure 1). Alternatively, extensive pneumatization may extend into the orbital roofs, posteriorly into the skull base to the clinoid processes, and into pterygoid plates (Figure 2).

The most common diseases of the paranasal sinuses are inflammatory or infectious. Inflammatory diseases of the sinuses are a leading cause of loss of productivity both at work and at school, although they typically are not serious and respond promptly to appropriate medical management. An estimated 32.3 million people in the United States have chronic sinusitis. Additionally, approximately 10% of the population suffers from allergic sinus disease. The cost of treating sinus disease runs into the billions of dollars, without taking into account loss of work or the additional costs incurred in a diagnostic work-up. Given the trend toward "rationed" medical care, physicians are increasingly working toward an effective means of both early diagnosis and follow-up in these patients. This includes documenting disease as well as recognizing and imaging patients who will require surgery.

The radiologists' paradigm of sinonasal imaging has undergone extensive revision over the last 5 years, from cheap, easily accessible, but relatively low-accuracy plain-film radiography, to the current use of third- and fourth-generation computed tomography (CT) and high field-strength (1.5 tesla) magnetic resonance (MR). Diagnosing sinus pathology previously required interpretation of subtle shadows, loss of contours, and other indirect signs from the visualized sinuses on those plain-film studies. This technique not only was insensitive for disease detection, but also was grossly inadequate for staging or accurately following subtle changes of the diseased sinus. Sinus CT and MR have allowed us to directly visualize the pathology within the sinuses, as well as depict the normal anatomy. Though often nonspecific, these tools are an immense improvement over plain-film sinus depiction, and can give a reliable reproducible baseline for comparison on subsequent examinations.

Recent advances in the last decade have occurred not only in imaging the paranasal sinuses, but also in treating chronic sinusitis with the development and wide acceptance of functional endoscopic sinus surgery (FESS). In FESS, the otolar-

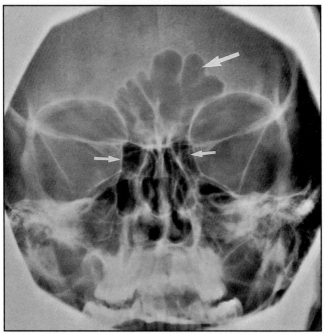

Figure 3: Example of normal paranasal sinuses on plain-film radiograph. Modified Caldwell's view demonstrating the frontal sinuses (large white arrow) and portions of the ethmoid sinuses (small white arrows).

yngologic surgeon removes bony portions of both the paranasal sinuses and the nasal vault. This preserves the mucociliary clearance system while reestablishing normal sinus drainage pathways.

We rely on the primary care physician to refer patients with chronic or recurrent symptoms to the otolaryngologist, who can then determine which patients will be candidates for FESS. This decision is complex, and although imaging helps make that decision, it is not made on the imaging findings alone. FESS performed on patients with near-normal or even normal CT images is not without precedent or justification. Computed tomography in the coronal plane (the same orientation used in FESS) provides the endoscopic sinus surgeon with a road map in performing sinus surgery to maximal efficacy and safety. Computed tomography, in combination with nasal endoscopy, is the most effective method of diagnosing surgical disease.

The following sections review the use of diagnostic imaging in the evaluation of the sinuses in patients with acute inflammatory and chronic inflammatory disease. In addition, we will review concerns about radiation and imaging intensive care unit and pediatric patients, and touch on several emerging imaging techniques.

Sinus Plain Films

The traditional imaging examination of the paranasal sinuses has been plain-film radiography. Sinus plain-film radiography consists of a series of radiographs to depict the sinuses in orthogonal planes, using a standard x-ray tube and a film-screen combination. The normal sinus anatomy depicted on plain-film radiography is shown in Figure 3. Plain-film radiography of the sinuses has recently received much attention because of concerns about cost constraints and outcome-based imaging. Should a clinician image with CT or MR if the clinically relevant question can be answered with the less expensive plain-film examination? Sinus x-rays are predictive of maxillary sinusitis, and perform reasonably well in diagnosing frontal and sphenoid sinusitis (Figure 4). However, they are less reliable in depicting abnormalities in the ethmoid sinuses, which are often the first affected in sinus inflammatory disease. Plain films are not only poor in documenting the presence of disease, but also less specific and sensitive than sinus CT in depicting the extent of sinus abnormalities. One study plainly concluded that sinus radiographs were not reliable enough to be integral to the clinical decision process. Thus, the use of plain radiographs of the sinuses has clearly been reduced by medical cost-containment concerns, by replacement with superior techniques, and by its own obvious weaknesses.

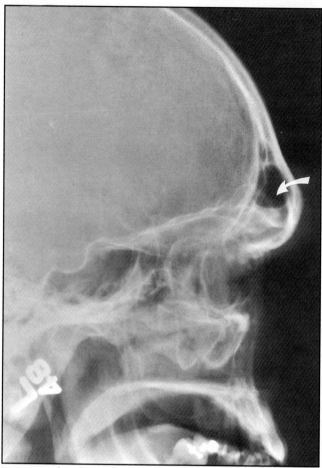

Figure 4: Plain-film example of sinusitis. Lateral radiograph demonstrating air-fluid level within the frontal sinus (curved white arrow). The posterior wall of the frontal sinus appears intact.

Computed Tomography

X-ray computed tomography has proven to be invaluable in the evaluation of the paranasal sinuses. Newer-generation

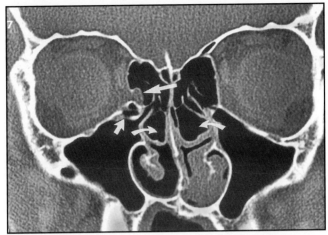

Figure 5: Coronal CT of the sinuses at the level of the ostiomeatal complex. Note the presence of bilateral pneumatized middle turbinates (concha bullosa) (curved white arrows). There is a Haller air cell (infraorbital ethmoid air cell) on the right (short straight arrow). An important finding is the dehiscence of the thin medial wall of the orbit on the right, with the herniation of fat medially out of the orbit (long straight arrow). The surgeon must be alerted to this finding if this patient were a candidate for functional endoscopic surgery to avoid potential orbital complications.

scanners can provide, within a few minutes, high-resolution axial images of tissue slabs that are only millimeters thick. The primary strengths of sinus CT imaging are improved contrast resolution, ie, ability to depict bone, bone-air, and bone-soft tissue interfaces; and spatial resolution, ie, ability to depict very small structures. We wish to gain numerous pieces of information from imaging the patient with inflammatory sinus disease. This information includes the status of the bony walls, the nature of material within the sinuses, and the status of adjacent normal structures such as the orbit, brain, and midface. The status of the bony walls of the sinuses is important both in benign sinus disease as well as in

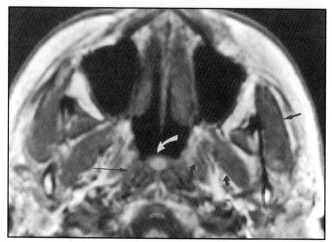

Figure 6: Axial T1-weighted MRI. Note the excellent soft-tissue contrast with delineation of the masseter (short black arrow), pterygoid (short curved black arrows), and longus colli (thin long black arrows). Incidental note is made of a Tornwaldt's cyst (curved white arrow).

sinus neoplasms (Figure 5). Computed tomography is markedly superior to plain-film radiography in depicting soft-tissue structures adjacent to or within the paranasal sinuses, although it is not as capable as MR in soft-tissue distinction. Despite this relative weakness, CT remains less expensive than MR and typically more available. Computed tomography has multiplanar capability in patients who can tolerate the coronal position within the gantry. The direct view of the sagittal plane is not possible; however, it is obtainable through 3-D reformation.

Magnetic Resonance Imaging (MRI)

The superior soft-tissue contrast obtained with MR is well known (Figure 6). Previously, the inability to obtain thin sections with MR had been a relative problem. However, with current-generation scanners and improved coils, MR can now obtain high-resolution images of slice thickness less than or equal to present CT scanners. Three-dimensional acquisitions also can be performed with the ability to postprocess and manipulate the data set, allowing depiction in any conceivable plane.

The lack of signal from bone in aerated sinus cavities causes problems, and with susceptibility artifacts, even thin amounts of soft-tissue signal adjacent to either bone or air may be inapparent. We still find performing MR difficult on patients with claustrophobia, though newer "open" magnets are being promoted to alleviate this concern. Additionally, there are various contraindications to MR. Patients with implanted biomedical devices (eg, cardiac pacemakers, vascular clips), or metallic foreign bodies in the eyes, cannot undergo MR. Patient cooperation is key in obtaining diagnostic MR images. Pediatric patients can pose special problems, many of whom will require the added risk of sedation to obtain a diagnostic study.

Ultrasonography

Ultrasonography (US) of the sinuses has been used in Europe, typically as a confirmation of the presence of free fluid in the sinuses in acute sinusitis. Ultrasonography is as attractive as it is portable, does not use ionizing radiation, and is relatively inexpensive when compared to CT and MR. However, because the ultrasound beam must penetrate a bone interface, there are limits to its depth of penetration. This seriously lessens the utility of US in detecting the presence or extent of disease. Operator dependence can be extremely variable, and can limit both the achievement of diagnostic-quality images and the ability to determine whether the condition has worsened or improved. The examination is limited to the frontal and maxillary sinuses, excluding the ethmoid and sphenoid sinuses. It has no place in the diagnosis of other sinus inflammatory or neoplastic processes, and has seen little use in the United States.

Imaging Acute Sinus Inflammatory Disease

Sinusitis is the most prevalent complication of the common cold seen in general and emergency medical departments. The sensitivity and specificity of diagnosing sinusitis in the absence of radiographic findings, however, is low; many patients with "sinus" headaches or histories of congestion may not have radiographic findings consistent with sinusitis. Maxillary toothache has a high sensitivity, but low specificity (<20%), while sinus tenderness has poor sensitivity and specificity (45% and 65%, respectively). A recent study of five independent clinical predictors of sinusitis demonstrated that the overall clinical impression (ie, gestalt) was more accurate than any single historic factor or physical finding.

What ancillary methods are reliable in increasing the diagnostic confidence in a patient with probable sinusitis? From the standpoint of imaging, the choices are few. Transillumination is a relatively low-tech imaging method for sinuses, used by some practitioners with relative confidence. It is considerably operator-dependent, and again limited in the sinuses that can be visualized. Plain-film radiography remains a commonly requested examination, both by otolaryngologists and other clinicians. As described earlier, plain-film examinations have real limits, and should not be accepted as any sort of gold standard. Limited CT examinations may have some utility, and can be quite accurate as long as the involved sinus is depicted. Patients presenting to the otolaryngology department at the University of Virginia with suspected acute sinusitis will undergo a thorough history and physical examination, occasionally including a flexible nasal endoscopic examination. The clinical decision to treat or not to treat is then made. If the differential diagnosis remains unclear, an imaging study is recommended. We emphasize that this represents only a small subset of the patients presenting with sinus complaints.

The typical patient presenting with facial pain that is maximal over a sinus, purulent nasal discharge ipsilateral to the involved sinus, headache, or constitutional symptoms probably does not need sinus films or a CT to confirm the diagnosis. However, not all patients are so easily categorized, and some degree of uncertainty in diagnosis is not uncommon. We do not advocate the routine performance of a complete sinus series in these patients. A single Waters' projection of the sinuses can be reviewed with the radiologist and confirm acute sinusitis fairly often. Treatment can then begin, or additional views taken if necessary. A limited plain-film examination such as this may provide some additional information, despite the limits in evaluating the ethmoid sinuses. However, even a limited CT examination unquestionably has superior diagnostic efficacy.

Some institutions have variations on a limited CT examination, offering a series of fewer than 10 images, with coronal and axial views, and with a corresponding low cost comparable to a plain-film series of the sinuses. A discussion with the radiology staff at the referral institution can help determine the possible examinations that may be appropriate for the clinical situation. Clinicians should be aware, however, that positive CT findings do not always correspond to acute bacterial infection. Up to 40% of asymptomatic patients may have some degree of sinus opacification. Additionally, a recent study by Gwaltney and Phillips et al reported that a large percentage of patients with recent onset of common cold symptoms show abnormal CT findings, 79% of which resolved in 2 weeks without antibiotic therapy. Moreover, patients with sinonasal polyp disease may also demonstrate sinus opacification on CT in the absence of clinical signs of infection (Figure 7). These drawbacks of imaging specificity underscore the importance of relating the history and physical examination to the imaging examination. Follow-up CT scans in a patient diagnosed with acute sinusitis may be necessary if response to treatment is delayed or if complications are suspected. However, CT is not indicated each time symptoms recur.

Imaging Complications
of Acute Sinus Inflammatory Disease

Complications of sinusitis, although uncommon in the postantibiotic era, can be life-threatening. In patients treated for acute sinusitis, the onset of swelling, facial numbness,

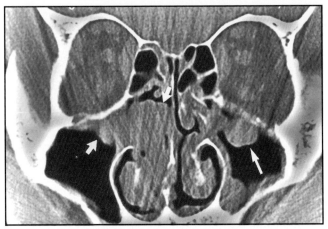

Figure 7: Coronal CT image of the sinuses demonstrating polypoid soft-tissue density in the left maxillary sinus (long white arrow). A conglomerate soft-tissue density extends through the ostium of the right maxillary sinus and into the nasal vault (short white arrows). This process extended posteriorly to the area of the choana (not shown). This patient did not show clinical signs of sinusitis, and on endoscopy was found to have an antrochoanal polyp on the right, with other polyps in the left maxillary sinus.

ocular dysfunction, or proptosis should prompt a search for extrasinus (eg, orbital, intracranial) extension (Figure 8), as well as other complications of sinusitis (eg, pyocele, mucocele, fungal sinusitis, underlying neoplasm) (Figure 9). In these patients, additional plain-film radiography is not indicated, and either CT or MR examination is mandated. Magnetic resonance has become the imaging tool of choice in complications of paranasal inflammatory disease, whether they be orbital, intracranial, or deep-facial spread.

Chronic and Recurrent Sinus Inflammatory Disease

Chronic sinusitis has been defined as sinusitis symptoms lasting more than 12 weeks. This time course connotes an ir-

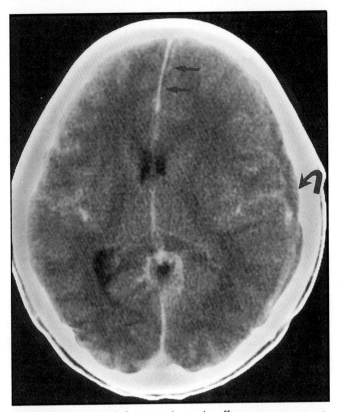

Figure 8: Patient with fever and nasal stuffiness, now presenting with altered consciousness. Because of the patient's altered mental status, a contrast-enhanced CT was performed through the brain that demonstrated an extra-axial fluid collection on the left (curved black arrow). The patient was immediately taken to the operating room, where a subdural empyema was found. Note the shift of the falx to the right (short black arrows).

reversible epithelial injury of the sinus mucosa. Nasal endoscopy has recently been advocated as the primary step in the work-up for these patients.

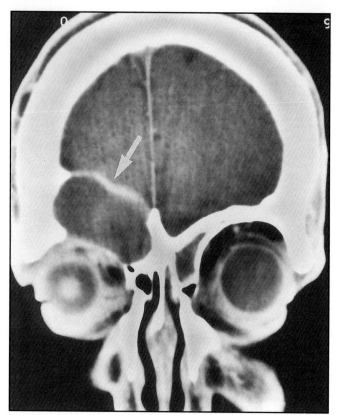

Figure 9: Patient presenting with proptosis on the right. Contrast-enhanced coronal CT demonstrates a homogenous expansile soft-tissue density within the right frontal sinus (large white arrow). Note the dehiscence of bone over the superior aspect of this mass.

When endoscopy fails to explain the patient's symptoms, imaging should be used. Patients with chronic or recurrent sinus symptoms, or with significant sinonasal polyposis, will simply not benefit from plain-film examination. Likewise, much has been written on the difficulty of depicting chronic sinus inflammatory disease with MRI, notably the desiccated concretions or coexistent fungal infections that may exist in chronically obstructed or diseased sinuses. Fungal disease or chronic sinus concretions may be missed entirely on MRI (Figure 10). Computed tomography is more accurate in diagnosing fungal sinus disease, and can depict concretions within the sinuses that will be inapparent on MR (Figure 11). In these patients, as well as patients with sinonasal polyposis, we believe that coronal screening sinus CT is adequate if the disease is confined to the nasal cavity and paranasal sinuses.

Pre-FESS Imaging

The decision to perform FESS is typically made before the performance of an imaging examination, based on an appropriate clinical history (eg, chronic sinusitis, recurrent acute sinusitis, sinonasal polyposis). However, use of this surgical technique in acute sinusitis may gain in acceptance. The goal of the imaging examination in these patients is to provide the surgeon with superior anatomic detail. Simply imaging an acutely ill patient and depicting extensive sinonasal abnormalities may confirm a diagnosis. However, the lack of good anatomic landmarks, of demineralization of cartilage or bone adjacent to an active inflammatory process, and of extensive mucosal abnormalities, hinder the road map of the anatomy that can be encountered after treatment of the acute infection and the shrinkage of acutely inflamed mucosa. Coronal high-resolution thin-section sinus CT has become widely accepted as necessary to the preoperative evaluation of patients undergoing FESS (Figure 12). We have slightly modified the original technique described by Zinreich, with wide acceptance from our referral otolaryngology colleagues. We also strive to improve the quality of the examinations by insisting on a medical "tune-up" before sinus imaging, to maximize the anatomic detail obtained. The importance of patient preparation in this group has previously been discussed. Patients at the University of Virginia undergo maximal medical therapy to address acute infections, shrink inflamed mucosal membranes, and reduce hyperplastic mucosa. One or multiple

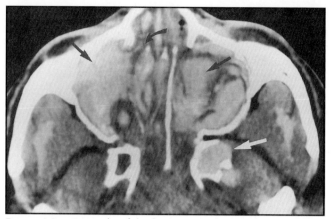

Figure 10a: Example of the limitations of MRI of the sinuses. Axial CT in a patient with polyposis demonstrates complete opacification of the maxillary sinuses with hyperdense material (black arrows). Note extension into and expansion of the left pterygoid plates (white arrow).

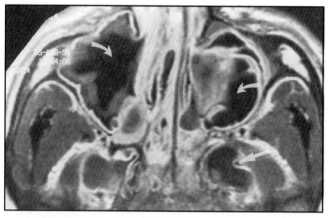

Figure 10b: Axial T1-weighted image at the same level demonstrates absence of signal (curved white arrows) within the maxillary sinuses and within the left pterygoid plates (white arrow). These areas could be mistaken for normal air-filled regions, underestimating the degree of disease.

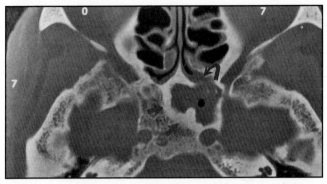

Figure 11: Patient with chronic sinus complaints. Axial CT at the level of the sphenoid sinus demonstrates opacification of the sphenoid sinus, with soft-tissue density material blocking the sinus ostium (curved black arrow). This is a chronic process, given the degree of bony sclerosis and thickening involving the walls of the sphenoid sinus (short black arrows).

courses of antibiotics, nasal corticosteroids, decongestants, antihistamines (reserved for allergic patients), and nasal saline washes are prescribed for 3 to 4 weeks before a screening sinus CT. We have used the prone coronal position in all patients who can tolerate it. The supine, or "hanging head" coronal position may be used, but free fluid, if present in the maxillary sinuses, will tend to move toward the maxillary sinus ostia and obliterate them.

A modern continuously rotating CT or spiral CT can be performed in less than 5 minutes. No intravenous contrast is needed. The scan technique, though low (150 mA, resulting in low radiation exposure), generates image contrast that is diagnostic for definition of anatomic structures. These images are adequate for evaluation of various densities within the sinus contents, which can indicate fungal sinus disease or concretions within the sinuses. Though some clinicians advocate additional windowing to increase sensitivity for extrasinus pathology, it has not been our routine. If there is concern for orbital pathology, intracranial pathology, or other extrasinus

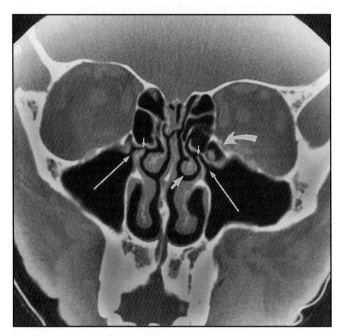

Figure 12: Normal anatomy on routine screening sinus CT. Coronal CT obtained to show the ostiomeatal complex. Note the ostia of the maxillary sinuses (long white arrows) and the uncinate processes (small white arrows). A large Haller cell (ethmoid air cell extending laterally into the orbital floor) is present on the left (curved white arrow). A paradoxically curved middle turbinate is present on the left (short thick white arrow). Note how the normal middle turbinate on the right curves laterally as it courses caudally.

complications, we will add axial images, administer intravenous contrast, or request MR.

We do not believe that a limited CT scan consisting of several axial and coronal images is adequate for pre-FESS planning. We also do not believe that a screening sinus CT as performed with this protocol is appropriate for headaches, complications of acute sinusitis, nonspecific sinonasal complaints, etc. Computed tomography is a tailored and specific examination for a particular indication, namely the preoperative evaluation of a patient undergoing FESS. As this technique enables us to perform the CT relatively quickly, we have been able to reduce the charge for an examination.

As MR becomes more refined, we may be approaching a time when it may prove acceptable as an alternative to screening sinus CT, or may even prove superior. Ignoring the susceptibility problems, we still require both a high spatial resolution to image the complex anatomy of the lateral nasal wall, and contrast resolution to allow adequate depiction of the bone, cartilage, and mucosal surfaces of the nasal cavity and sinuses. These are only now becoming more available by MR.

Imaging the Pediatric Patient

Children average eight upper respiratory illnesses per year, compared to two to three per year for adults. The incidence of sinusitis in children is 5% to 13%. As in adults, imaging should be reserved for cases in which the differential diagnosis is uncertain. Imaging is also becoming the primary method in chronic and recurrent cases, because nasal endoscopy requires a great deal of patient cooperation, and therefore is difficult to perform in the pediatric population.

In the normal development of the paranasal sinuses, the maxillary sinuses are not visible on plain radiographs until 8 to 12 weeks of age, the ethmoids at 3 to 6 months, the sphenoid at 3 years, and the frontals at 8 to 10 years. Accordingly, adequate correlation between sinus opacification and clinical symptoms is not present until at least 2 years of age. Consequently, some clinicians recommend sinus imaging only in children older than 7 years, or in children older than 2 years with suspected severe disease.

Plain films of the sinuses in children can be misleading. Using CT as the gold standard, plain films have had a false-negative rate of 45% and a false-positive rate of 35% in infants and children. With these discouraging numbers, it is clear that the choice of plain films is fraught with error. Computed tomography, while offering improved sensitivity and specificity, has its own drawbacks, namely: higher cost; increased radiation exposure; and the frequent necessity of sedation to properly perform the examination. Even with the drawbacks of plain-film radiography, some clinicians still advocate it for diagnosing and managing pediatric patients with medically treated sinus disease. We contend that even in the pediatric population, the benefits of a good-quality limited CT examination continue to outweigh the drawbacks of the plain-film examination. Complicated sinusitis is best evaluated with a contrast-enhanced CT in both the axial and coronal planes, with MR reserved to delineate intracranial extension.

Radiation

Imaging the pediatric population with x-rays immediately raises concern about radiation exposure. Much improvement has been made in recent years in CT dosimetry. The finely collimated beam used in thin-section CT, and the increased sensitivity of radiation detectors, have allowed the radiologist to significantly reduce the technique necessary to provide high-quality images, and subsequently reduce the radiation exposure to the patient. However, even reduced dosage CT entails greater radiation exposure than that of plain-film radiography, with the lens and thyroid being primary organs of concern. The dose delivered by screening sinus CT is approximately 17.6 mGy for a technique of 210 mA. We have decreased this exposure by using a technique of 150 mA. This results in a far less dosage than the single dose of 2 Gy or fractional doses of 4 Gy needed to produce cataract formation, and the 2- to 2.5-Sv dose to double the human mutation rate. As long as the study is clinically indicated, there are no exposure limits for medical radiation. However, it remains prudent to use an x-ray or CT examination only when the results will alter clinical management.

Future Developments in Sinus Imaging

New developments in MR may uncover additional and unique information about the nasal cavity and paranasal sinuses. While limits can be measured to evaluate air movement within the nasal cavity or resistance to normal flow, no imaging study can now depict normal or abnormal airflow. Investigators at several institutions, including the University of Virginia, are working with gases, which can achieve significant paramagnetic properties through irradiation with a laser, and can serve as a contrast agent for MR. Helium may prove optimal for this use because it is not significantly absorbed and has good signal-to-noise properties. Lung images have been obtained with xenon and helium, and visualization of the proximal airways is a consistent feature. We hope to soon visualize the actual passage of a gas bolus through the nasal cavity, and learn the pattern of air exchange within the paranasal sinuses. Patients with acute sinus inflammatory disease, posttrauma patients, sleep apnea patients, asthmatic and upper-airway reactive disease patients, and numerous other patient populations may be study material for this new technology.

Newer surgical techniques are also being developed that use computer-assisted stereotactically guided endoscopic equipment. These promise to make complicated as well as routine cases safer, and may improve surgical outcomes, although this has yet to be shown.

Summary

The contribution of imaging to the management of both benign and malignant sinus and nasal cavity disease is significant. Close working relationships among the primary care physician, the otolaryngologist, and the head and neck radiologist are essential for optimal patient management. Though we now have powerful tools for the evaluation of the sinonasal region, new emerging technologies will likely further our knowledge of this complex and somewhat poorly understood region, and allow us the ability to use imaging in ways never before envisioned.

Suggested Readings

Braams JW, Pruim J, Freling NJ, et al: Detection of lymph node metastases of squamous-cell cancer of the head and neck with FDG-PET and MRI. *J Nucl Med* 1995;36:211-216.

Dolan RW, Chowdhury K: Diagnosis and treatment of intracranial complications of paranasal sinus infections. *J Oral Maxillofac Surg* 1995;53:1080-1087.

Friedman WH, Katsantonis GP, Bumpous JM: Staging of chronic hyperplastic rhinosinusitis: treatment strategies. *Otolaryngol Head Neck Surg* 1995;112:210-214.

Gliklich RE, Metson R: The health impact of chronic sinusitis in patients seeking otolaryngologic care. *Otolaryngol Head Neck Surg* 1995;113:104-109.

Goodman GM, Martin DS, Klein J, et al: Comparison of a screening coronal CT versus a contiguous coronal CT for the evaluation of patients with presumptive sinusitis. *Ann Allergy Asthma Immunol* 1995;74:178-182.

Guarderas JC: Rhinitis and sinusitis: office management. *Mayo Clin Proc* 1996;71:882-888.

Lund VJ, Kennedy DW: Quantification for staging sinusitis. The Staging and Therapy Group. *Ann Otol Rhinol Laryngol Suppl* 1995;167:17-21.

Maclennan AC: Radiation dose to the lens from coronal CT scanning of the sinuses. *Clin Radiol* 1995;50:265-267.

Maclennan AC, McGarry GW: Diagnosis and management of chronic sinusitis. Do not rely on computed tomography. *Br Med J* 1995;310:529-530.

Middleton H, Black RD, Saam B, et al: MR imaging with hyperpolarized 3He gas. *Magn Reson Med* 1995;33:271-275.

Phillips CD, Platts-Mills TA: Chronic sinusitis: relationship between CT findings and clinical history of asthma, allergy, eosinophilia, and infection. *AJR Am J Roentgenol* 1995;164:185-187.

Ramadan HH: Endoscopic treatment of acute frontal sinusitis: indications and limitations. *Otolaryngol Head Neck Surg* 1995; 113:295-300.

Reuler JB, Lucas LM, Kumar KL: Sinusitis. A review for generalists. *West J Med* 1995;163:40-48.

Roberts DN, Hampal S, East CA, et al: The diagnosis of inflammatory sinonasal disease. *J Laryngol Otol* 1995;109:27-30.

Shankar L, Evans K, Hawke M, et al: *An Atlas of Imaging of the Paranasal Sinuses*. Singapore, Imago Publishing LTD, 1994.

Wald ER: Radiographic sinusitis: illusion or delusion? *Pediatr Infect Dis J* 1993;12:792-793.

Schwartz RB: Helical (spiral) CT in neuroradiologic diagnosis. *Radiol Clin North Am* 1995;33:981-995.

Shapiro MD, Som PM: MRI of the paranasal sinuses and nasal cavity. *Radiol Clin North Am* 1989;27:447-475.

Sillers MJ, Kuhn FA, Vickery CL: Radiation exposure in paranasal sinus imaging. *Otolaryngol Head Neck Surg* 1995;112:248-251.

Som PM, Curtin HD: Chronic inflammatory sinonasal diseases including fungal infections. The role of imaging. *Radiol Clin North Am* 1993;31:33-44.

Som PM, Curtin HD, eds. *Head and Neck Imaging*. St. Louis, Mosby-Year Book, 1996, pp 65-69.

Wagner W: Changing diagnostic and treatment strategies for chronic sinusitis. *Cleve Clin J Med* 1996;63:396-405.

Wippold FJ 2nd, Levitt RG, Evens RG, et al: Limited coronal CT: an alternative screening examination for sinonasal inflammatory disease. *Allergy Proc* 1995;16:165-169.

Chapter 7

Nosocomial Sinusitis, Fungal Sinusitis, and Sinusitis in the Immunocompromised Patient

B acterial and fungal sinusitis are well recognized as complications of systemically immunocompromised patients, as well as those with transnasal tubes (eg, nasogastric and respiratory intubation). This chapter will briefly address nosocomial sinusitis, fungal sinusitis, and sinusitis associated with human immunodeficiency virus (HIV) infection.

Nosocomial Sinusitis

Bacterial sinusitis has been thought to be a cause of fever, sepsis, and, occasionally, death in critically ill patients with nasal cannulas. Most patients with nosocomial sinusitis are in an intensive care unit (ICU). Obstruction of the ostiomeatal complex (OMC) by mucosal edema associated with trauma from a transnasal foreign body seems logical. As also expected, the longer a foreign body is in place, the greater likelihood of sinusitis. Patients with a history of sinus problems are more likely to have problems with transnasal tubes, but most patients who have 7 days of intranasal tube placement will have radiographic evidence of maxillary sinus abnormalities. However, studies of the transnasal puncture-obtained fluid from the maxillary sinus is usually free of microorganisms. In some cases, this may be from antimicrobial therapy the patient is receiving for other reasons.

Although it is clear that nosocomial bacterial sinusitis can result in intracranial infections, septicemia, bronchopneumonia, and thoracic empyema, it is surprising that these complications are not common. The exception is bronchopneumonia. In one carefully done study, 67% of 43 maxillary sinusitis patients developed bronchopneumonia, with 38% of those having the same bacteria found initially in maxillary sinus aspirates as in subsequent lower respiratory tract secretions.

Computed tomography scans are more likely to demonstrate sinusitis than are plain x-rays. Pneumatic otoscopy has been reported to be useful as a screening tool, but may not be generally available. Surprisingly, "sterile" or infectious paranasal sinusitis is *not* commonly associated with occult fever or other infectious complications in critically ill ICU patients.

Most of the definitive microbiologic studies on nosocomial sinusitis have come from France, where transnasal aspiration of maxillary sinus fluid is commonly performed. This is rarely done now in the United States; therefore, antimicrobial therapy is largely empiric. Many patients are already receiving antimicrobial treatment when diagnosed with presumed bacterial sinusitis. The change to or addition of agent(s) active against nosocomial respiratory tract pathogens in a particular ICU would be prudent. *Pseudomonas aeruginosa*, *Staphylococcus aureus*, and anaerobes should be covered.

A review of the limited literature on nosocomial sinusitis suggests the following:

(1)   Transnasal endotracheal and gastric tubes in patients with previously normal maxillary sinuses are associated with more than 90% occurrence of radiographic maxillary sinus involvement after 7 days.

(2)   If endotracheal and gastric tubes are placed in the oropharynx, the incidence of radiographic maxillary sinus involvement drops to less than 25%.

(3)   The risk factors for maxillary sinusitis are greatest with a nasal endotracheal tube in place.

(4)   Infectious maxillary sinusitis associated with a nasal endotracheal tube is frequently associated with bronchopneumonia.

(5)   Although fever and complications of nosocomial sinusitis occur, they are not common.

(6)   Computed tomography scan of the sinuses should be taken to evaluate intubated patients with fever and signs of sepsis from unknown origins.

(7)   Further work needs to be done regarding the positioning of patients and the use of nasal constrictors in ICUs to assure better sinus drainage.

(8)   Patients believed to have nosocomial sinusitis should be evaluated by an otolaryngologist who can perform rhinoscopy and pneumatic otoscopy.

(9)   Management of the patient with nosocomial sinusitis, especially in the ICU, usually does not require surgery.

(10)   Sinusitis is an important nosocomial infection in critically ill patients, and its prevention may protect against the development of bronchopneumonia.

Fungal Sinusitis

Fungal sinusitis is uncommon. When it occurs, it may be a slowly evolving process or, in immunocompromised patients, rapidly progressive and even fatal (Figure 1). Patients with severe immunocompromise secondary to aggressive treatment for malignancy, AIDS, bone marrow and solid organ transplantation, and uncontrolled diabetes mellitus represent a high-risk group for serious sinusitis, including fungal sinusitis. Despite prolonged antimicrobial therapy for many problems, including repeated episodes of bacterial sinusitis, fungal sinusitis is uncommon in otherwise normal patients, even though fungi are ubiquitous in dust, plants, decaying organic matter, and soil. Nevertheless, a fungal cause should be considered in any patient with chronic or life-threatening sinusitis. Fungi enter the nasal and paranasal sinus mucosa from inhaled dust particles. Most inhaled fungi produce no problems, but there are case reports of most mycotic genera associated with sinusitis. *Aspergillus*, *Phycomycetes* (*Mucor*, *Rhizopus*) and black molds (phaeohyphomycosis such as *Alternaria*) are most common. Interestingly, *Candida* rarely causes sinusitis (or pneumonia), despite readily infecting the oral and esophageal mucosa.

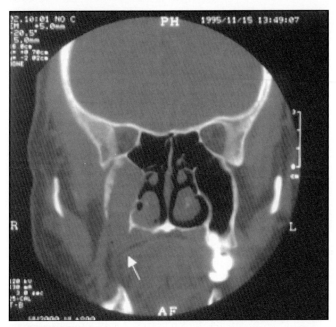

Figure 1: Maxillofacial CT showing total opacification of the right maxillary sinus with destruction of the bony floor and portions of the medial wall caused by zygomycosis.

Aspergillus Sinusitis

Aspergillus species (*fumigatus*, *flavus*, and *niger*) are the most common causes of fungal sinusitis. *Aspergillus* can cause three disease states: (1) allergy; (2) mycetoma; and (3) invasive aspergillosis. Allergic *Aspergillus* sinusitis is similar to allergic *Aspergillus* bronchopulmonary disease. Presumably, the entrance of *Aspergillus*-contaminated dust particles to the sinus mucosa allows the fungal antigen to react with IgE-sensitized mast cells, initiating the allergic-immunologic cascade. The process produces thickened polypoid mucosa with gelatinous, brownish or green-black material with concretions. Patients present with nasal obstruction and greenish discharge that persist despite antibacterial therapy. Imaging studies reveal sinus opacification, but some bony erosion may also be seen, suggesting malignancy. If the nasal secretions contain eosinophils, and septated hyphae with 45-degree angle branching can be seen with Gomori's methenamine silver (GMS) stain, allergic *Aspergillus* sinusitis is the most likely diagnosis. Phaeohyphomycosis (*Bipolaris*, *Curvularia* species, etc) can produce the same allergic reaction in the sinuses, and they also have septated hyphae. Culture is necessary to establish which fungus is the culprit, but is usually negative. The initial treatment is the same.

Treatment consists of surgical débridement of the involved sinuses with removal of all affected mucosa, as well as relief of septal obstruction and other areas of blockage. Itraconazole (Sporanox®) is being studied for the treatment of allergic *Aspergillus* bronchopulmonary disease. If it is effective in that setting, it should be effective for allergic *Aspergillus* sinus disease as well. Itraconazole is also active in vitro against phaeohyphomycosis.

Aspergillus mycetoma occurs in the immunocompetent patient with chronic sinusitis. In this disease, *Aspergillus* will not actually invade the sinus mucosa. It may produce a mycetoma or "fungus ball" that can remain in the sinus, gradually enlarging and even causing erosion of bone. On CT scan, *Aspergillus* mycetoma has a characteristic appearance. Mycetoma must be totally removed, along with any diseased mucosa. Sinus drainage is mandatory. Instillation of amphotericin B (Fungizone®), 1 mg/mL sterile water, into the involved sinus may be employed.

Aspergillus-induced sinus infection in severely immunocompromised patients may invade sinus mucosa and adjacent bone, as well as spread to the proximal soft tissues. These patients are usually very neutropenic or have depressed T-cell function. Patients may be septic and the process may progress rapidly, resembling rhinocerebral mucormycosis. The patients are critically ill from the combination of their underlying disease and the fungal infection. They commonly have headache, fever, cough, and dark, bloody nasal discharge. These patients require immediate evaluation by an infectious disease consultant, otolaryngologist, and ophthalmologist.

Treatment consists of radical surgical débridement of all involved tissue, as well as high-dose liposomal amphotericin B (5 to 7 mg/kg/d). Granulocyte colony-stimulating factor (GCSF) and granulocyte macrophage colony-stimulating factor (GMCSF) are promising in helping the patient's own defenses.

Phycomycetes (Zygomycosis, Mucormycosis) Sinusitis

Mucor, *Rhizopus*, and *Absidia* are the most common causes of rhinocerebral mucormycosis. This large, nonseptated fungus rarely produces invasive disease unless the patient is *markedly* immunocompromised. Patients with diabetic ketoacidosis, leukemia with granulocytopenia, hemochromatosis, and those on high-dose corticosteroids constitute most patients who develop mucormycosis. The fungus invades blood vessels, causing obstruction with fungal mycelia resulting in infarction. This produces the classic black necrosis seen on intranasal examination. Ophthalmologic findings are common. The process spreads intracranially very rapidly from the sinuses, and infarction of an eye is not unusual. Once intracranial extension occurs, the mortality rate is greater than 50%. Therefore, early suspicion of diagnosis and rapid treatment are mandatory.

The therapy for mucormycosis requires consultation as soon as possible with an infectious disease specialist, neurosurgeon, ophthalmologist, and otolaryngologist. As in invasive aspergillosis, adequate débridement of all infarcted necrotic tissue must be performed. It is not uncommon for patients to require further débridement. Careful daily examinations are necessary. In addition to surgery, high-dose liposomal amphotericin B (5 to 7 mg/kg/d) should be started as soon as the diagnosis is suspected. Granulocyte macrophage colony-stimulating factor, 250 mg subcutaneously daily as long as the white blood cell count does not exceed 25,000/mm^3, has been used. Because *Phycomycetes* thrive in an oxygen-poor environment, hyperbaric oxygenation has been suggested as an adjuvant treatment. Unfortunately, hyperbaric chambers are not available to most physicians.

Sinusitis in HIV-Infected Patients

Although it was recognized early that paranasal sinus problems are common in patients with HIV infection, the pathophysiology remains unclear. HIV infection is associated with aberrant immunologic responses, especially if AIDS is present. There is an increased incidence of both allergic and bacterial sinusitis in HIV-infected patients. High IgE levels are frequently found, and correlate with severe sinusitis. There may be IgG subclass deficiencies, such as low IgG2. As in patients without HIV, maxillary and ethmoid sinuses are more often involved than frontal or sphenoid. Both cigarette smoking and intranasal cocaine are potential aggravating factors.

The microbial agents that cause sinusitis in the general population are common in HIV-infected patients because response is defective to encapsulated bacteria such as *Streptococcus pneumoniae*, *Haemophilus influenzae*, and *Moraxella catarrhalis*. At least 30% of pneumococcal disease in HIV patients is attributable to sinusitis. Patients receiving trimethoprim/sulfamethoxazole (TMP/SMX) for prophylaxis against *Pneumocystis carinii* who develop sinusitis are likely to have TMP/SMX-resistant microorganisms. Staphylococci, *P aeruginosa* (17% in one study), and *Aspergillus* are more frequent in HIV patients with sinusitis.

Sinusitis should always be considered in the HIV-infected patient with fever with or without headache, especially if AIDS is present. A high index of suspicion is necessary to make an early diagnosis in this patient population. As in nosocomial sinusitis in the ICU, radiologic abnormalities of the sinuses are the rule in HIV-infected patients who are symptomatic.

When an antimicrobial agent is chosen for empiric therapy, ciprofloxacin (Cipro®), 750 mg q 12 h, remains the agent of choice because of its activity against the encapsulated organisms, as well as *P aeruginosa* and most methicillin-sensitive staphylococci. If the patient does not respond to empiric therapy, cultures should be obtained from the OMC to identify unusual or resistant organisms such as *Cytomegalovirus*, *Mycobacterium avium-intracellulare*, *Microsporidia*, and *Aspergillus*. The length of antimicrobial therapy for infectious sinusitis in HIV patients is the same as for those without HIV infection. Although most patients will partially respond to antimicrobial therapy, complete resolution of clinical findings is unusual, presumably because of the allergic component. Nevertheless, antihistamines are contraindicated for bacterial sinusitis because thickening of secretions may occur. In fact, guaifenesin has been recommended for chronic rhinosinusitis in HIV patients to decrease mucus viscosity and theoretically improve mucociliary clearance. Systemic decongestants benefit some patients. The role of intranasal corticosteroids is not clear. Patients who do not readily respond to therapy should be evaluated by an otolaryngologist and an infectious disease specialist.

Interestingly, surgical drainage is rarely performed for bacterial sinusitis associated with HIV infection, despite the observation that medical management is frequently difficult, especially as the patient's immune status decreases. We hope that with the availability of highly active antiretroviral therapy, sinusitis in HIV-infected patients will occur less often, and be less severe when it does.

Summary

Failure of an HIV-infected patient to respond to bioavailable antibacterial therapy and achieve relief of obstruction with bacterial sinusitis implies: (1) that surgery is indicated; (2) the presence of a resistant bacterium such as methicillin-resistant *S aureus*; (3) the presence of a nonbacterial pathogen, such as a fungus; (4) chronic allergic sinus disease; or (5) a nonspecific sinusitis associated with HIV infection.

Suggested Readings

Corey JP, Delsupehe KG, Ferguson BJ: Allergic fungal sinusitis: allergic, infectious, or both? *Otolaryngol Head Neck Surg* 1995;113:110-119.

de Shazo RD, Chapin K, Swain RE: Fungal sinusitis. *N Engl J Med* 1997;337:254-259.

Del Borgo C, Del Forno A, Ottaviani F, et al: Sinusitis in HIV-infected patients. *J Chemother* 1997;9:83-88.

Gross CW, Becker DG, eds: The Otolaryngologic Clinics of North America. Advances in Sinus and Nasal Surgery. Philadelphia, WB Saunders, vol 30, June 1997.

O'Donnell JG, Sorbello AF, Condoluci DV, et al: Sinusitis due to *Pseudomonas aeruginosa* in patients with human immunodeficiency virus infection. *Clin Infect Dis* 1993;16:404-406.

Rouby JJ, Laurent P, Gosnach M, et al: Risk factors and clinical relevance of nosocomial maxillary sinusitis in the critically ill. *Am J Respir Crit Care Med* 1994;150:776-783.

Chapter 8

Antimicrobial Therapy

Antimicrobial therapy is useful in the management of bacterial sinusitis when used in conjunction with relief of obstruction and with other appropriate therapy. As of November 1997, the FDA had approved seven antimicrobial agents for the treatment of bacterial sinusitis in adults. They are:

- Amoxicillin/clavulanate (Augmentin®) 500/125 mg q 8 h or 875/125 mg q 12 h for "sinusitis caused by β-lactamase-producing strains of *Haemophilus influenzae* and *Moraxella (Branhamella) catarrhalis.*"

- Cefprozil (Cefzil®) 250-500 mg b.i.d. for "acute sinusitis caused by *Streptococcus pneumoniae*, *Haemophilus influenzae* (beta-lactamase-positive and -negative strains) and *Moraxella catarrhalis* (including beta-lactamase-producing strains)."

- Cefuroxime axetil (Ceftin®) 250 mg b.i.d. for "acute bacterial maxillary sinusitis caused by *Streptococcus pneumoniae* or *Haemophilus influenzae* (non-beta-lactamase-producing strains only)."

- Ciprofloxacin (Cipro®) 500 mg b.i.d. for 10 days for "acute sinusitis caused by *Haemophilus influenzae*, *Streptococcus pneumoniae*, or *Moraxella catarrhalis.*"

- Clarithromycin (Biaxin®) 500 mg b.i.d. for "acute maxillary sinusitis due to *Haemophilus influenzae*, *Moraxella catarrhalis,* or *Streptococcus pneumoniae.*"

Table 1: FDA-Approved Package Insert In Vitro Microbiologic Activity

	S pneumoniae			H influenzae	
	Penicillin-sensitive	Penicillin-intermediate	Penicillin-resistant	Beta-lactamase (-)	(+)
Amoxicillin/clavulanate	+	+	0	+	+
Azithromycin	+	0	0	+	+
Cefprozil	+	0	0	+	+
Cefuroxime axetil	+	0	0	+	+
Ciprofloxacin	+	0	0	+	+
Clarithromycin	+	0	0	+	+
Doxycycline	+	0	0	+	+
Levofloxacin	+	0	0	+	+
Loracarbef	+	0	0	+	+
Sparfloxacin	+	+	+	+	+
Trimethoprim/sulfamethoxazole	+	0	0	+	+

- Loracarbef (Lorabid®) 400 mg q 12 h for "acute maxillary sinusitis caused by *Streptococcus pneumoniae*, *Haemophilus influenzae* (non-beta-lactamase-producing strains only) or *Moraxella catarrhalis* (including beta-lactamase-producing strains)."
- Levofloxacin (Levaquin®) 500 mg q.d. orally or IV for "acute maxillary sinusitis due to *Streptococcus pneumoniae*, *Haemophilus influenzae*, or *Moraxella catarrhalis*."

Table 1 lists in vitro antibacterial activity for the approved as well as commonly used agents for bacterial sinusitis.

Antimicrobials that are being considered by the FDA for approval for the treatment of bacterial sinusitis include

| M catarrhalis | | S aureus | | Oral anaerobes |
Beta-lactamase (-)	(+)	Methicillin-sensitive	Methicillin-resistant	
+	+	+	0	+
+	0	+	0	some
+	0	+	0	+
+	+	+	0	some
+	+	+	0	0
+	+	+	0	some
+	+	+	0	some
+	+	+	0	0
+	+	+	0	+
+	+	+	0	0
0	0	0	0	0

azithromycin (Zithromax®), 500-mg initial dose followed by 250 mg daily for 4 days, and sparfloxacin (Zagam®), 400-mg initial dose followed by 200 mg once daily for 9 days. In addition, several generically available antimicrobial agents that have been frequently and reliably used for the treatment of acute bacterial sinusitis have not been approved by the FDA for this indication. They include ampicillin (500 mg every 6 hours), amoxicillin (500 mg every 8 hours), doxycycline (Doryx®, Vibramycin®, 100 mg every 12 hours) and trimethoprim/sulfamethoxazole (Bactrim™, Septra®, 160/800 mg every 12 hours). The emergence of penicillin-resistant bacterial sinus pathogens has rendered ampicillin and amoxicillin

---

Table 2: Antimicrobials That Should Not be Used Alone for Bacterial Sinusitis

- Clindamycin (no *H influenzae* or *M catarrhalis* activity)
- Erythromycin (no *H influenzae* activity)
- Ofloxacin (levofloxacin more active and convenient)
- Tetracycline (doxycycline safer and more convenient)

---

less useful. Orally administered antimicrobials that do not have a place in the empiric management of ambulatory patients with bacterial sinusitis are listed in Table 2.

No antimicrobial agent has been approved for use in *chronic* bacterial sinusitis or acute bacterial exacerbations of chronic sinusitis; however, the choice of antibiotic is no different than that for acute bacterial sinusitis. We treat patients with acute exacerbations of chronic bacterial sinusitis for 21 to 28 days rather than the usually recommended 10 to 14 days for acute sinusitis. If there is any sign of maxillary dental problems, suspicion of anaerobes rises in the patient with chronic sinusitis, making an agent with antianaerobic activity preferable.

Knowledge of the antimicrobial susceptibility pattern of the organisms most likely to be associated with community-acquired bacterial sinusitis in your geographic area is necessary in choosing empiric therapy. Because beta-lactamase-producing strains of *H influenzae* and *M catarrhalis* are common in certain areas of the United States, ampicillin, amoxicillin, cefuroxime axetil, and loracarbef would not be first-choice agents. If the clinician is concerned about intermediate penicillin-resistant *S pneumoniae*, amoxicillin/clavulanate, cefprozil, ciprofloxacin, doxycycline, and levofloxacin are better choices for the outpatient with bacterial sinusitis. If bacterial sinusitis is related to maxillary dental disease, anaerobes are more likely to be involved, and amoxicillin/clavulanic acid or doxycycline would be good choices for oral therapy.

Because safety is always a primary concern when treating an outpatient, a caveat includes possible phototoxicity associated with doxycycline and sparfloxacin. However, in general, all the agents used in treatment of bacterial sinusitis are well tolerated. Doxycycline does not accumulate in the presence of decreased renal function, which is common in elderly patients (see Table 3 for comparison of antimicrobials used to treat ambulatory patients with presumed bacterial sinusitis).

If convenience of administration is important, then amoxicillin/clavulanate 875/125 mg b.i.d., doxycycline 100 mg b.i.d., cefuroxime axetil 250 mg b.i.d., ciprofloxacin 500 mg b.i.d., loracarbef 400 mg b.i.d., cefprozil 500 mg b.i.d., and clarithromycin 500 mg b.i.d. are reasonable. Azithromycin, levofloxacin, and sparfloxacin require administration only once daily.

The bioavailability (absorption) of doxycycline and the fluoroquinolones is markedly affected by divalent and trivalent cations such as calcium, magnesium, iron, zinc, etc. Therefore, if these are taken within 2 hours of levofloxacin or sparfloxacin administration, the antimicrobial effect may be diminished by 50% or more for the entire 24 hours, because these agents are given only once daily.

It is extremely difficult to separate mild bacterial sinusitis from viral rhinosinusitis in the first week of a common cold. Some patients are obviously overtreated. If antimicrobial therapy is believed appropriate for this type of patient, the best initial agents are clearly either doxycycline or trimethoprim/sulfamethoxazole for the nonpregnant female. Doxycycline and trimethoprim/sulfamethoxazole are also the least expensive agents available (less than $1.00 per day). Duration of therapy is very controversial, but earlier studies have shown that bacteria persist in large amounts in the sinus after symptoms have resolved. Therefore, we favor 14 days of antimicrobial therapy when its use is elected. Long-term follow-up studies with varying lengths of therapy are needed to settle the issue. Clinicians should encourage patients to take all the medication in the prescription and not save any in the medicine cabinet for the next episode.

Table 3: Oral Agents for Ambulatory Patients With Bacterial Sinusitis

Efficacy (≥85%)	Use in Pregnancy*	Least Major Side Effects
All	Amoxicillin/ clavulanate	Azithromycin
		Cefprozil
	Azithromycin	Cefuroxime axetil
	Cefprozil	Ciprofloxacin
	Cefuroxime axetil	Doxycycline
		Levofloxacin
	Loracarbef	Loracarbef

* All agents Category B-no teratogenic effects in nonhuman animals.

Patients who fail to respond to initial antimicrobial therapy for bacterial sinusitis should have a limited computed tomography (CT) scan taken of the sinuses. A consultation with an otolaryngologist may be beneficial. The specialist usually will perform an endoscopic evaluation and obtain a specimen for culture and sensitivity. If the CT scan shows no fluid accumulation that would require surgical drainage, a change of antibiotic should be considered. Good second-line agents include amoxicillin/clavulanate, azithromycin, ciprofloxacin, clarithromycin, levofloxacin, and sparfloxacin.

If the patient presents with a fever up to 101°F associated with facial pain, including maxillary toothache, with or without edema and erythema over the maxillary sinus, a blood culture and endoscopic swab of the ostiomeatal com-

Least Food/Drug Interactions	Once-Daily Dosage	Least Expensive
Amoxicillin/ clavulanate	Azithromycin	Doxycycline
	Levofloxacin	Trimethoprim/ sulfamethoxazole
Azithromycin (tablet)	Sparfloxacin	
Cefprozil		
Cefuroxime axetil		
Clarithromycin		
Loracarbef		

plex (OMC) are indicated. This would allow for subsequent isolation of potentially resistant pathogens. The patients in this category need careful follow-up. Empiric treatment for these adult patients includes 2 g of ceftriaxone (Rocephin®) as a single IM dose followed by high-dose amoxicillin/ clavulanic acid (875/125 q 8 h). A limited CT scan of the sinuses should be performed if the patient has not improved within 24 hours. If the patient is allergic to penicillin, an oral fluoroquinolone should be considered using the doses cited previously.

Problems arise when patients with clinical sinusitis are severely ill and have evidence of central nervous system or orbital involvement. These patients need an emergency head CT and surgical consultation. Vancomycin (Vancocin®) and

Table 4:	Initial Empiric Antimicrobial Treatment Recommendations for Bacterial Sinusitis
Mild	Doxycycline or trimethoprim/sulfamethoxazole
Moderate	Amoxicillin/clavulanate, azithromycin, or ciprofloxacin
	Consider initially giving ceftriaxone 2 g IM as a single dose
Severe	Vancomycin IV plus ceftriaxone IV
	If beta-lactam allergic: vancomycin IV plus chloramphenicol IV, or ciprofloxacin IV, or trimethoprim/sulfamethoxazole IV

ceftriaxone should be started as soon as possible after obtaining blood cultures. This will ensure adequate coverage of highly penicillin-resistant *S pneumoniae* and beta-lactamase-producing *H influenzae* and *M catarrhalis,* as well as methicillin-resistant *Staphylococcus aureus*, and most gram-negative enteric bacilli and gram-positive anaerobes that might be associated with polymicrobic infection. If the patient has a history of anaphylaxis caused by a beta-lactam antibiotic, ceftriaxone should be replaced with an agent with good central nervous system penetration such as chloramphenicol (Chloromycetin®), or trimethoprim/sulfamethoxazole. Surgical drainage should be performed as needed.

The roles of *Mycoplasma*, *Chlamydia,* and *Legionella* as causes of sinusitis have been inadequately studied. We assumed in the past that these pathogens were not important because most patients responded to ampicillin or amoxicillin. Nevertheless, these organisms would be adequately covered with the use of azithromycin, ciprofloxacin, clarithromycin, doxycycline, or levofloxacin. The presence of unusual organisms isolated from sinus aspiration or from the OMC (*P aeruginosa, Aspergillus*, etc) frequently requires consultation with an infectious-disease specialist to help choose the most appropriate antimicrobial therapy.

No studies have supported any vaccine use to prevent bacterial sinusitis. However, after the patient recovers from bacterial sinusitis, we administer pneumococcal vaccine and yearly influenza vaccine, regardless of the patient's age. If the patient is 65 years of age or older, we also give a single dose of *H influenzae* type b conjugated vaccine, since it is recognized that the antibody titer against *H influenzae* type b falls with aging. One problem is that most of the *H influenzae* strains are untypeable and, if not encapsulated, would not be expected to respond to antibodies generated against *H influenzae* type b capsular polysaccharide. Obviously, the best preventive measure for bacterial sinusitis would be an effective vaccine or therapy for the viruses that cause the common cold. Quitting smoking will improve host defenses that fight infection.

Important Considerations

- Viral rhinosinusitis is common and cannot be clinically distinguished from bacterial sinusitis.
- Viral rhinosinusitis responds to placebo just as well as to antibacterials, ie, it is self-limiting.
- Antimicrobials may be beneficial to patients with viral rhinosinusitis whose nasopharyngeal secretions contain *H influenzae*, *M catarrhalis,* or *S pneumoniae*.
- If a patient is still ill after 1 week of presumed viral rhinosinusitis, antimicrobial therapy plus a decongestant is beneficial.
- The appropriate length of antimicrobial therapy has not been established for acute bacterial sinusitis. Three to 21 days of therapy have been used, with many experts recommending 10 to 14 days for an initial episode, and longer therapy for patients with acute exacerbations of chronic sinusitis.

- The agents effective for acute bacterial sinusitis are also effective for acute bacterial exacerbations of chronic sinusitis; however, the prevalence of anaerobic bacteria in the latter is increased.
- For patients with mild bacterial sinusitis, therapy with doxycycline or trimethoprim/sulfamethoxazole is reasonable. For those with moderately severe disease, all of the oral agents listed in Table 1 should be adequate, but amoxicillin/clavulanate, azithromycin, or one of the listed fluoroquinolones is preferred. The use of a single IM injection of ceftriaxone on initial visit has not been studied, but we favor this in moderately severe cases where outpatient therapy is elected. Patients who are ill enough to be hospitalized should receive empiric parenteral antimicrobials pending appropriate culture and sensitivity studies. These may include vancomycin and ceftriaxone, or in the case of severe beta-lactam allergy, vancomycin IV plus chloramphenicol IV, or ciprofloxacin IV, or trimethoprim/sulfamethoxazole IV (Table 4).
- Overall, the efficacies of the oral agents listed in Table 1 do not really differ. Therefore, other factors, such as previous therapy, cost, convenience, potential drug interaction problems, and safety, and antimicrobial resistance patterns are important in deciding which agent to use for empiric therapy for bacterial sinusitis.

Suggested Readings

Joshi N, Miller DQ: Doxycycline revisited. *Arch Intern Med* 1997;157:1421-1428.

Donald TJ, Gluckman JL, Rice DH: *The Sinuses*. New York, Raven Press, 1995.

Chapter 9

Medical Therapy

Once the diagnosis of sinusitis is made, medical therapy is instituted. Therapies vary depending on the underlying cause of sinusitis. The underlying cause may be any precursor of rhinitis. These include upper respiratory infection; seasonal or perennial allergies; eosinophilic nonallergic rhinitis; vasomotor rhinitis; aspirin intolerance; tumors; atrophic rhinitis that may be rhinitis medicamentosa caused by overuse of topical nasal decongestants; rhinitis secondary to pregnancy; hypothyroidism; Horner's syndrome; and Wegener's granulomatosis. Anatomic causes may be foreign body; nasal polyps; nasal septal deviation; turbinate hypertrophy; and enlarged tonsils and adenoids. Functional etiologies include immune deficiency, immotile cilia, and cystic fibrosis. These differential diagnoses should be kept in mind during history taking and physical examination. Medical therapy also differs between acute and chronic sinusitis.

The ethmoid sinuses and the ostiomeatal complex (OMC) are usually involved in cases of recurrent and chronic sinusitis and, therefore, therapy is aimed at relieving obstruction of the OMC, in addition to treating any present infection. When this obstruction is obviously anatomic (eg, secondary to deviated nasal septum, extensive sinonasal polyps, or tumor), early surgical intervention may be necessary. In most instances, however, medical therapy is instituted before considering surgical therapy, and even when surgery is performed, medical therapy should be continued to achieve good long-term results.

The medical management of sinusitis may include one or more of the following: antibiotics, topical decongestants, systemic decongestants, topical nasal corticosteroids, nasal lavage or saline nasal spray, humidification, mucolytics, antihistamines, cromolyn, and immunotherapy.

Medical Management of Acute Sinusitis

The treatment of acute sinusitis includes antibiotics, decongestants, nasal lavage or saline spray, and an optional topical nasal corticosteroid.

Antibiotics

Ten to 14 days of antibiotic therapy are recommended for patients with acute sinusitis. The microorganisms most frequently seen in acute community-acquired sinusitis are *Streptococcus pneumoniae* and *Haemophilus influenzae*. See Chapter 8 for appropriate antibiotic choices.

Decongestants

For treatment of acute sinusitis, the topical decongestant oxymetazoline (Afrin®), 2 puffs in each nostril b.i.d. for 3 to 5 days, provides rapid and effective vasoconstriction. This decreases the obstruction of boggy turbinates and decreases the inflammation that obstructs the OMC. Prolonged use of topical decongestants (>5 days) can lead to rebound congestion or rhinitis medicamentosa. Pediatric-strength oxymetazoline frequently works well in adults and has less rebound congestion. If the congestion associated with acute sinusitis lasts longer than 3 days, oral decongestants such as pseudoephedrine hydrochloride, 30 to 60 mg b.i.d. or q.i.d., should be used.

Nasal Lavage/Saline Nasal Spray

Saline nasal spray or irrigation is recommended to cleanse thick secretions from the nose and sinuses. This simple, eco-

Table 1: Medical Management of Acute Sinusitis

- Antibiotics (10-14 days)
- Topical decongestant (no longer than 5 days)
- Oral decongestant (if necessary after discontinuing topical decongestant)
- Nasal lavage or saline nasal spray
- Humidification (cool-mist humidifier, steamy showers, 8 full glasses of water per day)
- Mucolytic (if desired to thin secretions)
- Topical nasal corticosteroid usually not necessary
- Antihistamines are *not* recommended

nomical treatment is effective, but unfortunately is under-used. Saline nasal spray is available over the counter as sterile physiologic saline solution in a squeeze-type spray bottle. Alternatively, saline solution may be prepared at home with half a teaspoon of salt dissolved in 8 oz warm tap water. A pinch of baking soda may be added. The patient should place the solution in a spray bottle or ear bulb syringe for lavage. Two to 4 puffs of saline nasal spray should be administered at least t.i.d. The alternative, more aggressive method is lavage with a bulb syringe while leaning over the sink with the mouth open. Repeated full syringe wash and aspiration is recommended at least 3 times daily to wash out the secretions if they cannot be effectively removed with saline spray alone.

Humidification

Humidification of inspired air and hydration are other methods recommended to clear thick secretions. A cool-mist humidifier, hot steamy showers, and ingestion of at least 8 full glasses of water per day are effective.

Topical Nasal Corticosteroids

For most episodes of acute sinusitis, the patient responds adequately to the above measures without the need for a topical nasal corticosteroid. However, topical nasal corticosteroids become very important in the management of chronic or allergic rhinitis, recurrent acute sinusitis, and chronic sinusitis.

Antihistamines

Antihistamines, in general, should not be used to treat acute suppurative sinusitis. Patients with sinusitis must avoid antihistamines because they potentially thicken the secretions and lead to crust formation, which can further obstruct the OMC. However, antihistamines can be quite helpful in profuse rhinorrhea that is obviously the result of allergic rhinosinusitis. Table 1 outlines the agents used in the medical management of acute sinusitis.

Medical Management of Chronic Sinusitis

The mere presence of chronic sinusitis or recurrent acute sinusitis warrants referral to a specialist. The otolaryngologist will perform a comprehensive evaluation, considering all possible underlying etiologies for the sinusitis. Depending on the history and examination, immunologic and allergic workups also may be necessary.

Chronic sinusitis is treated similarly to acute sinusitis, with some slight differences. Treatment includes an antibiotic, a topical nasal corticosteroid, an oral decongestant, nasal lavage or saline spray, humidification, and a mucolytic (Table 2). In chronic sinusitis, antibiotics are recommended for 3 to 4 weeks, and topical nasal corticosteroids are recommended on a long-term basis. Antihistamines are not recommended unless there is an obvious underlying allergic etiology.

Antibiotics

In addition to the common pathogens (*S pneumoniae*, *H influenzae*, *Moraxella catarrhalis*) associated with acute sinusitis, chronic sinusitis is associated with greater *Staphylococcus aureus* and anaerobic species. Therefore, amoxicillin is not considered first-line treatment for chronic sinusitis. Rather,

> **Table 2: Medical Management of Chronic Sinusitis**
>
> - Antibiotics (at least 21 to 28 days)
> - Topical nasal corticosteroid (regular daily use)
> - Oral decongestant
> - Nasal lavage or saline nasal spray
> - Humidification (cool-mist humidifier, steamy showers, 8 full glasses of water per day)
> - Mucolytic
> - Antihistamines are *not* generally recommended unless allergic etiology is known

greater broad-spectrum coverage is required. Antibiotics are recommended for at least 21 to 28 days in chronic sinusitis. See Chapter 8 for appropriate antibiotic choices.

Topical Nasal Corticosteroids

Topical nasal corticosteroids, along with antibiotics, are considered primary therapy for chronic sinusitis. While antibiotics treat the infectious component of sinusitis, topical nasal corticosteroids treat the inflammatory component, thereby reducing edema and obstruction of the OMC. Several safe preparations are available. These agents are highly active topically, with the ability to remain in tissues because of their high lipid solubility. The small amounts that are absorbed systemically are rapidly metabolized by the liver and, therefore, no systemic side effects are expected at the recommended doses. These drugs include beclomethasone dipropionate (Vancenase®, Beconase®), flunisolide (Aerobid®, Nasarel™), triamcinolone acetonide (Nasacort®), budesonide (Rhinocort®), and fluticasone (Flonase™).

In contrast to the topical decongestants, which should not be used for more than 5 consecutive days, the topical nasal corticosteroids are considered safe for chronic use. Subjects should be advised to be patient because the topical nasal corticosteroids have a delayed onset of action with clinical improvement expected after 7 to 10 days. The patient must understand that they are not effective on a haphazard, as-needed basis, and that these corticosteroids require regular daily administration. Most of the preparations are dosed as 2 puffs in each nostril daily. Beconase® and Nasarel™ are currently administered b.i.d. The maximum recommended dosage should be used for at least the first 4 weeks to control symptoms, and otolaryngologists and allergists often continue this dosage for 2 months or longer. The dosage may be weaned to 1 puff in each nostril daily when symptoms are well controlled.

Many of the topical nasal corticosteroids are available as aerosol or aqueous preparations. Regardless of preparation, local side effects may include burning, irritation, sneezing, dryness, crusting, bleeding, and, very rarely, septal perforation. Many physicians feel that the local side effects are reduced with aqueous preparations. Certainly, patients who complain of nasal dryness should be offered the aqueous type. These patients should also increase the use of nasal saline. The choice of the delivery system often depends on physician or patient preference. All patients should be instructed to avoid spraying medially toward the septum to reduce the risk of these local side effects.

Decongestants

Because the treatment of chronic sinusitis requires a more prolonged course than acute sinusitis, topical decongestants are not recommended. When they are used for more than 5 days, topical decongestants can lead to rhinitis medicamentosa, which will only make matters worse. Instead, oral systemic decongestants such as pseudoephedrine and phenylpropanolamine are used during the full course of treatment.

Nasal Lavage/Saline Nasal Spray

Daily frequent use of nasal lavage or saline nasal spray is recommended for chronic sinusitis. This is administered on a chronic basis in the same manner described for acute sinusitis.

Humidification

Humidification with a cool-mist humidifier, frequent hot steamy showers, and consumption of 8 full glasses of water per day are all recommended.

Mucolytics

The most common mucolytic agent is guaifenesin. This has long been used and is considered effective as a mucolytic and expectorant in bronchitis. Guaifenesin is considered effective in liquefying the annoying thick secretions associated with chronic sinusitis. Guaifenesin is the most common expectorant found in cough syrups. For chronic sinusitis, the recommended daily dose is 2,400 mg. This is available in tablet or liquid form, and may also be found in combination with oral decongestants. In higher doses, guaifenesin acts as an emetic, and occasionally the dose used in chronic sinusitis must be limited because of GI discomfort.

Antihistamines

As in acute sinusitis, antihistamines are not recommended as standard treatment in chronic sinusitis because of their significant drying effects that can lead to crusts and stasis of secretions. However, if the patient has a significant history of underlying allergies, antihistamines may be necessary to help control the allergic response. Table 2 outlines the medical management of chronic sinusitis.

Medical Management of Allergic Rhinosinusitis

An estimated 20% of the U.S. population suffers from allergic disease. The nose is most commonly affected in the allergic individual. Symptoms include sneezing, pruritus (eyes, nose, palate, and throat), watery eyes, rhinorrhea, congestion, cough, and postnasal discharge. An estimated 40 million Americans are afflicted with allergic rhinitis, which in turn predisposes to many cases of sinusitis.

Allergic rhinitis is a hypersensitivity of the sinonasal mucosal membranes to allergens, mediated through IgE antibodies. Allergic rhinitis may be classified as seasonal or perennial. Allergic rhinitis is considered seasonal when the symptoms occur only during specific periods of the year, depending on exposure to pollens. Ragweed, trees, and grasses are the most common sources of seasonal allergens. Allergic rhinitis is considered perennial when the symptoms occur for more than 2 hours per day for more than 9 months. Dust mites, molds, and animal dander represent the most common sources of perennial allergens.

Avoidance

Avoidance is one therapeutic measure to prevent allergic symptoms. If the allergen is known (eg, cat dander), then avoidance of exposure will be effective. However, multiple allergens often are responsible. Allergy testing may provide clearer identification of the allergens to be avoided. Environmental control measures should be taken to eliminate such culprits as dust mites and mold. When avoidance is difficult or unsuccessful, pharmacotherapy and immunotherapy are treatment options.

Pharmacotherapy

Pharmacotherapy for the allergic patient includes antihistamines, decongestants, cromolyn sodium, and corticosteroids.

Antihistamines

Antihistamines are important in the treatment of inhalant allergies. Antihistamines work by competing with histamine for H_1 binding sites in respiratory mucosa. Histamine is a mediator of anaphylactic reactions and immediate allergic reactions. Antihistamines work to prevent these reactions, and therefore are most effective when given before exposure to allergens.

Classes of antihistamines include the traditional first-generation antihistamines, and newer, second-generation antihistamines. Antihistamines are effective in relieving symptoms such as itching, sneezing, rhinorrhea, and postnasal drip. The primary side effect of the traditional antihistamines is sedation. They can also cause significant dryness and crusting

Table 3: Medical Management of Allergic Rhinosinusitis

- Avoidance of known allergens (inhalants and food)
- Environmental controls
- Antihistamines
- Decongestants
- Cromolyn sodium
- Corticosteroids
- Immunotherapy

within the nose. The second-generation antihistamines are considered nonsedating, and have less tendency to cause excessive dryness. Still, antihistamines should be avoided if possible during acute suppurative sinusitis because their drying action thickens the mucus and can exacerbate the condition.

Traditional antihistamines include diphenhydramine (Benadryl®), tripelennamine (PBZ®), chlorpheniramine maleate (Chlor-Trimeton®), meclizine (Antivert®, Bonine®), hydroxyzine (Atarax®), and promethazine (Phenergan®). Meclizine is useful for control of vertigo. Hydroxyzine is used as a tranquilizer, and promethazine is useful for control of nausea.

Second-generation antihistamines include terfenadine (Seldane®), astemizole (Hismanal®), loratadine (Claritin®), cetirizine (Zyrtec®), and fexofenadine (Allegra™). Terfenadine has lost popularity because of possible onset of ventricular arrhythmias when used concomitantly with ketoconazole (Nizoral®) and macrolide antibiotics. This potential also exists for astemizole. Astemizole has a rather long half-life (5 days for its parent compound and 3 weeks for its metabolites), which many clinicians find undesirable. Loratadine, cetirizine, and fexofenadine are the newest agents and seem to have no serious side effects. Loratadine and cetirizine are administered once daily, while fexofenadine is taken twice daily.

Decongestants

Decongestants are effective in combination with antihistamines in those allergic patients with associated nasal congestion. Decongestants can improve clinical efficacy in these patients by reducing swelling of the sinonasal mucosa by alpha-adrenergic-induced vasoconstriction. Many over-the-counter preparations combine antihistamines with decongestants. Seldane-D®, Claritin®-D, Claritin®-D 24, and Semprex™-D are second-generation antihistamines combined with a decongestant (pseudoephedrine) that are available by prescription. Semprex™-D is dosed up to 4 times daily. Seldane-D® and Claritin®-D are administered twice per day, and Claritin®-D 24 is administered once daily.

Cromolyn Sodium

Cromolyn sodium (Nasalcrom®) is available as a topical nasal spray that stabilizes mast cells, thereby preventing mast cell degranulation and preventing release of inflammatory mediators (eg, histamine, leukotrienes, thromboxanes, and prostaglandins). Cromolyn stabilizes mast cells by reducing calcium transport across cell membranes, thereby preventing the calcium-dependent degranulation process.

Cromolyn sodium is effective for both seasonal and perennial allergic rhinitis. It works for both acute and late-phase allergic reactions. Cromolyn sodium is most effective when taken before allergen exposure. It is effective neither for nonallergic sinusitis nor for the treatment of nasal polyps. Nasalcrom® is available as a spray pump. The dose is one spray in each nostril every 4 hours while awake. Relief of symptoms usually occurs within 4 to 7 days, after which the dose can be reduced to a maintenance level geared to the particular patient and continued throughout the allergen exposure period. Local and systemic side effects are minimal. Systemic absorption is less than 7%, with rapid renal and biliary excretion. Uncommon local side effects include sneezing, burning, and irritation.

Corticosteroids

Corticosteroids have an anti-inflammatory action that occurs by several mechanisms, including stabilization of lysosomal membranes, blockage of migratory inhibitory factor, and decrease in capillary permeability. Corticosteroids are administered either systemically or as topical nasal sprays. Because the topical nasal corticosteroids are quite effective for allergic rhinitis, systemic corticosteroids are rarely required. The topical nasal corticosteroid sprays are described in further detail earlier in this chapter.

For patients with mild or moderate allergies, adequate relief usually is obtained with appropriate avoidance and environmental controls, antihistamines, and either cromolyn sodium spray or topical nasal corticosteroid spray. Topical nasal corticosteroid spray is recommended for more persistent symptoms. Systemic corticosteroids are reserved for more severe cases. For patients who do not obtain satisfactory relief with avoidance and pharmacotherapy, immunotherapy may be effective.

Immunotherapy

The two recommended allergy testing options are serial end-point titration (SET) and radioallergosorbent test (RAST). Both SET and RAST give qualitative and quantitative information about the patient's response to specific allergens.

Serial End-Point Titration (SET)

Serial end-point titration (SET) requires serial skin applications of several dilutions of each antigen being investigated. When the patient is sensitive to a specific antigen, the wheal will increase by at least 2 mm with each increase in antigen dilution. The first dilution that leads to a 2-mm increase is the end point, which is considered the safe starting dose for immunotherapy for that specific antigen. Subsequently during immunotherapy, the clinical response determines changes in doses. Many clinicians who favor SET find that it has the advantage of providing immediate results. This allows immunotherapy to begin without any delay. The SET method involves testing suspected allergens based on the patient's history, therefore avoiding the need for a large in vitro test panel (as in RAST). SET is found to be quite sensitive. SET results can be affected by antihistamines, tranquilizers, and antidepressants. For example, antihistamines must be discontinued at least 48 hours before SET. Skin conditions may also alter results, because this method relies on skin application of antigen dilutions.

In Vitro Testing: Radioallergosorbent Test (RAST)

Radioallergosorbent test (RAST) involves taking a serum sample from the patient. An in vitro panel of allergens (antigens) is studied. Antigen-specific IgE antibodies present in the serum bind to allergens on a solid-phase paper disc. This is washed so only attached antibodies remain. These are then marked by binding radiolabeled antihuman IgE antibodies to the antigen-specific IgE antibodies. A scintillation counter then is used to measure the radiation count, which is directly proportional to the quantity of antigen-specific IgE antibodies from the serum sample. More recently, enzyme markers have replaced the radioactive labels. Results from RAST are then used to determine which allergens are responsible and guide immunotherapy. The results are also used to help calculate treatment doses. RAST has the advantage of greater comfort and ease of testing for the patient. The in vitro testing presents no risk of reaction to the patient. Medications and skin conditions will not affect RAST results. RAST is slightly less sensitive and more expensive than SET. Both SET and RAST give qualitative and quantitative information that may be used for immunotherapy. They can be safely applied in the office setting and are valuable in the treatment of allergic rhinosinusitis.

Food Allergy

Food allergy is increasingly recognized as a culprit in allergic disease. Cow's milk is the most common food allergen. Symptoms may be similar to those related to inhalant allergy. Cyclic and fixed food allergies may occur. The cyclic type is more common, representing approximately 95% of food allergies. Symptoms related to cyclic food allergy will occur several hours after ingesting the allergenic food. Fixed food allergies involve a type 1 immediate hypersensitivity reaction.

One method to test for food allergy is the deliberate oral challenge feeding test. First, the food is identified as suspect by noting its frequency in the diet diary. It is helpful to eliminate the suspect food throughout the 72 hours before administration of the oral challenge feeding test. Next, the food is ingested, and the patient is simply observed for the onset of allergic symptoms.

A second method to test food allergy is the provocative food test (PFT). Subcutaneous or intradermal injection of extract of the suspected food is performed. Onset of symptoms is expected within 30 minutes. These results correlate well with the results of oral challenge feeding tests.

Once a specific food allergy is determined, the main treatment is elimination of the food for at least 3 months. Often, the food may be slowly reintroduced after that time. Alternative treatment methods are injection or sublingual administration of a "neutralizing dose" of the food that is determined allergenic by PFT.

Allergies caused by inhalant allergens and food allergens certainly produce symptoms that can contribute to chronic sinus problems. Treatment options include careful identification and avoidance of suspected allergens; pharmacotherapy; and immunotherapy. Mild to moderate symptoms often can be controlled with environmental controls, antihistamines with or without decongestants, cromolyn sodium, and topical nasal corticosteroids. More severe symptoms may require more aggressive and prolonged medical therapy, testing with SET or RAST, and possible immunotherapy. Suspected food allergies also should be carefully identified and treated by elimination or injection technique.

Suggested Readings

Derebery MJ: Otolaryngic allergy. *Otolaryngol Clin North Am* 1993;26:593-611.

Druce HM: Adjuncts to medical management of sinusitis. *Otolaryngol Head Neck Surg* 1990;103:880-883.

Gwaltney JM Jr, Jones JG, Kennedy DW: Medical management of sinusitis: educational goals and management guidelines. The International Conference on Sinus Disease. *Ann Otol Rhinol Laryngol Suppl* 1995;167:22-30.

Kaliner MA, Osguthorpe JD, Fireman P, et al: Sinusitis: bench to bedside. Current findings, future directions. *J Allergy Clin Immunol* 1997;99:S829-S848.

King HC: Endpoint titration and immunotherapy. *Otolaryngol Clin North Am* 1985;18:703-717.

King HC: Diagnostic provocation testing and neutralization therapy for food allergy. In: Krause HF, ed. *Otolaryngic Allergy and Immunology*. Philadelphia, WB Saunders, 1989, pp 246-253.

King WP, Rubin WA, Fadal RG, et al: Provocation-neutralization: a two-part study. *Otolaryngol Head Neck Surg* 1988;99:263-277.

Mabry RL: Therapeutic agents in the medical management of sinusitis. *Otolaryngol Clin North Am* 1993;26:561-570.

Mabry RL: Pharmacotherapy with immunotherapy for the treatment of otolaryngic allergy. *Ear Nose Throat J* 1990;69:63-71.

Mabry RL: Topical pharmacotherapy for allergic rhinitis: new agents. *South Med J* 1992;85:149-154.

Mabry RL: Uses and misuses of intranasal corticosteroids and cromolyn. *Am J Rhinol* 1991;5:121-124.

Murray J: Topical nasal steroids. *Vanderbilt University Sinus Newsletter*, September 1996.

Nalebuff DJ: In vitro-based allergen immunotherapy. In: Krause HF, ed. *Otolaryngic Allergy and Immunology*. Philadelphia, WB Saunders, 1989, pp 163-168.

Nathan RA: Changing strategies in the treatment of allergic rhinitis. *Ann Allergy Asthma Immunol* 1996;77:255-259.

Stafford CT: The clinician's view of sinusitis. *Otolaryngol Head Neck Surg* 1990;103:870-874.

Willoughby JW: Serial dilution titration skin tests in inhalant allergy: a clinical quantitative assessment of biologic skin reactivity to allergenic extracts. *Otolaryngol Clin North Am* 1974;7:579-615.

Ziment I: Help for an overtaxed mucociliary system: managing abnormal mucus. *J Resp Dis* 1991;12:21-33.

Chapter 10

Surgical Management

S urgical management of sinusitis is indicated when: (1) medical management fails to relieve the patient of the bothersome symptoms of sinusitis; (2) the condition is associated with lower respiratory tract problems (eg, chronic bronchitis, asthma); and (3) complications of sinusitis are present or threatening. Traditional surgical procedures for the sinuses include the Caldwell-Luc operation, intranasal ethmoidectomy, frontoethmoidectomy, external ethmoidectomy, and transnasal ethmoidectomy. These procedures were designed to completely remove infection and the mucosal linings, leaving the sinuses without mucociliary function. We now know that normal mucociliary function is essential to the health of the paranasal sinuses.

In 1985, the use of nasal endoscopes for the diagnosis and surgical treatment of sinus disease was introduced and popularized in the United States. This brought dramatic change, as functional endoscopic sinus surgery (FESS) essentially replaced the traditional procedures for the surgical management of sinus disease. With nasal endoscopes, the narrow anatomic region of the ostiomeatal complex (OMC) can be visualized and accurately approached surgically. The combination of nasal endoscopy and computed tomography (CT) allows physicians to assess disease that previously went unrecognized.

The OMC, the small compartment located in the region between the middle meatus and the lateral nasal wall, represents the key region for drainage of the anterior ethmoid, maxillary, and frontal sinuses. Obstruction of the OMC causes a vicious cycle of events that leads to sinusitis. Ostiomeatal complex obstruction leads to mucosal congestion that decreases airflow and drainage. Secretions then thicken and become stagnant. Subsequently, mucosal gas metabolism changes result in hypoxia and damage to the cilia and epithelium. The environment becomes a culture medium for bacterial growth in the closed cavity. The retained secretions cause further tissue inflammation, and bacterial infection develops. Mucosal thickening causes further blockage of the OMC, completing the vicious cycle that will continue unless patency of the OMC is restored.

Sinus surgery using rigid nasal endoscopes has been developed as an approach termed *functional endoscopic sinus surgery* (FESS). The surgery is considered functional because it is a conservative approach aimed at restoring patency and normal mucociliary flow to the OMC (Figure 1). This allows for ventilation and drainage of the sinuses without destroying their normally functioning ciliated mucosal linings. The natural ciliary action can then clear secretions through the unobstructed ostia of the sinuses. Relieving obstruction of the OMC also provides access for topical nasal corticosteroids and saline application, which may be necessary for maintenance of healthy sinuses in certain individuals.

As nasal endoscopic techniques have advanced, the application of endoscopic surgery has expanded to include repair of choanal atresia, transnasal decompression of thyroid orbitopathy, repair of cerebrospinal fluid rhinorrhea, intranasal dacryocystorhinostomy, resection of skull base tumors, optic nerve decompression, and transsphenoidal hypophysectomy.

Procedures such as septoplasty and turbinate reduction often are combined with endoscopic sinus surgery, if indicated. These procedures may be performed either endoscopically or by traditional methods, depending on the surgeon's preference.

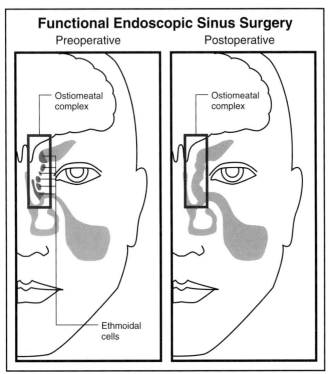

Figure 1: The preoperative and postoperative appearance of the ethmoid sinuses and the ostiomeatal complex in relation to functional endoscopic sinus surgery (FESS). Primary disease in the ethmoids and the OMC can lead to secondary sinusitis within the frontal and maxillary sinuses. FESS removes the diseased areas, thereby improving ventilation and drainage of the dependent sinuses. The mucosal lining usually returns to normal over time, making radical excision unnecessary.

Indications for Functional Endoscopic Sinus Surgery (FESS)

All patients who have recurrent acute sinusitis or chronic sinusitis should be referred to an otolaryngologist for nasal endoscopy and evaluation. The otolaryngologist can make an accurate diagnostic assessment based on history by nasal endoscopy combined with findings on CT scan of the paranasal sinuses. Any patient suspected of having significant allergic disease should be referred for work-up by an allergy specialist. In general, patients who fail medical therapy (see Chapter 9) are candidates for surgical management.

Indications in Recurrent Acute Sinusitis

Relative indications for FESS in adults and in children over 12 years old who have recurrent acute sinusitis include:
- 4 or more episodes of infection during the past 12 months;
- a trial of immunotherapy for allergic rhinosinusitis, or absence of allergy;
- presence of an anatomic variant, especially one causing OMC obstruction;
- prophylactic use of nasal corticosteroids, mucolytics, and decongestants.

Indications in Chronic Sinusitis

FESS is indicated in adults who have chronic sinusitis when there is endoscopic or CT scan evidence of sinusitis, and persistent disease despite at least 21 to 28 days of antibiotics. Endoscopic evidence may include polyps, mucosal hypertrophy, edema, and mucopurulent discharge from a sinus orifice. Decongestants, mucolytics, and nasal corticosteroids are recommended for the treatment of chronic sinusitis; if these are omitted from the medical regimen, the antibiotic therapy may fail. Allergy work-up and immunotherapy are recommended in individuals with significant allergies. Immunodeficiency and mucociliary dysfunction represent special situations. Patients with immunodeficiency may require immunoglobulin administration by an immunologist before considering FESS. Patients with mucociliary dysfunction who require surgery benefit from gravitational drainage of the sinus cavity (ie, large inferior meatus antrostomy), rather than FESS, which provides ventilation in the region of the middle meatus.

Anesthesia for FESS

FESS is performed in the operating room under either local anesthesia with intravenous sedation, or general anesthesia. This decision usually is based on patient or surgeon preference. Many physicians feel that local anesthesia and sedation results in less bleeding because of greater vasoconstriction. Those who support general anesthesia feel that blood pressure can be more easily maintained in a relatively hypotensive state to keep bleeding to a minimum. General anesthesia also prevents any movement of the patient during the procedure.

Regardless of whether IV sedation or general anesthesia is used, the nasal mucosa is decongested with topical oxymetazoline, phenylephrine, or cocaine. The lateral nasal wall is injected with lidocaine with epinephrine for hemostasis during the procedure. The lidocaine with epinephrine should be given at least 10 minutes before starting the procedure to take effect.

FESS Technique

Endoscopic sinus surgery is performed in either an anterior-to-posterior direction, or a posterior-to-anterior direction. The anterior-posterior technique is the more conservative approach referred to as FESS, and is best for limited disease that involves the anterior ethmoid, maxillary, or frontal sinuses. The posterior-anterior technique may be used for patients with pansinusitis, or in patients who have had prior sinus surgery that resulted in loss of anatomic landmarks.

Rigid nasal endoscopes are used to visualize the nasal cavity and lateral nasal wall. In general, 4-mm diameter rigid nasal endoscopes with 0-degree and 30-degree lenses are used. The procedure is begun with the 0-degree scope. The middle meatus is visualized. An incision is created in the mucosa just anterior to the uncinate process, and the uncinate process is removed. This exposes the ethmoid bulla, which represents the most prominent and anterior cell of the ethmoid sinuses. The ethmoid bulla is entered, and additional anterior ethmoid cells are removed, if necessary, back to the ground lamella.

The ground lamella, or basal lamella, represents the anatomic division between the anterior and posterior ethmoid cells. If CT scan suggests posterior ethmoid disease, the ground lamella is entered into the posterior ethmoid cavities. Posterior ethmoid cells are removed, if necessary, back to the sphenoethmoid recess. Extreme care is taken not to violate the ethmoid roof (fovea ethmoidalis), which separates the superior ethmoids from the cranial cavity. Extreme care also is taken not to violate the lamina papyracea, which is the paper-thin bone that separates the ethmoids from the orbit. Finally, normally appearing mucosal linings are maintained, rather than stripped out.

Once the ethmoidectomy is completed, the natural maxillary ostium is identified. If the maxillary sinus is involved, the ostium is enlarged to assure patency. Any secretions or polyps are removed from the sinus, with care taken to maintain mucosal linings. If the frontal sinus is involved, completion of anterior ethmoidectomy is confirmed and the frontal recess is cleared of any obstruction. The areas of the frontal recess and the maxillary ostium can be well visualized with the 30-degree rigid nasal endoscope. If there is sphenoid disease, the sphenoid ostium is located with the aid of the 0-degree endoscope, the ostium is enlarged, and any disease is removed.

The surgeon should address any further anatomic variants, such as nasal polyps or a concha bullosa. Concha bullosa is an aerated, enlarged middle turbinate that can cause obstruction of the OMC. Partial middle turbinectomy may be performed endoscopically to reduce the turbinate without narrowing the middle meatus, providing greater patency to the OMC. A deviated nasal septum may be repaired, or enlarged inferior turbinates may be reduced during FESS. These procedures may be performed endoscopically or by traditional techniques.

The posterior-anterior technique differs from anterior-posterior technique in that it begins in the sphenoid sinus and proceeds anteriorly through the ethmoid sinuses. Again, this technique is reserved for extensive pansinusitis or revision cases in which there has been loss of anatomic landmarks.

Powered Instrumentation

Powered instruments represent more recent advancements in endoscopic sinus surgery. The powered instruments were originally designed for endoscopic joint surgery and have been clearly established as essential tools for fine soft-tissue joint work in arthroscopic surgery. Smaller instruments were designed for temporomandibular joint surgery. They have become quite popular in sinus surgery because they offer the endoscopic surgeon greater technical precision. The powered instrument consists of a power source, a handpiece, and a disposable sheathed shaving cannula. Each shaving cannula has a blunt tip and a lateral aperture near the tip that faces 90 degrees. The shaver sucks soft tissue into the lateral aperture and subsequently "shaves" it with a rotating or oscillating inner blade. Because the blade is guarded, the instrument provides excellent control for precise resection of soft tissue without damaging surrounding tissues. Built-in suction continuously removes blood, secretions, and debris, and maintains a clear surgical field. The powered instruments offer the potential advantages of less trauma, decreased bleeding, shorter surgical time, greater comfort, improved recovery, and more rapid healing.

The most dramatic advantage of powered instrumentation has been seen in nasal polyps. Traditionally, nasal polyp surgery has been performed with manual instruments that work by avulsion of the polyps. This causes tearing of the tissues, which can include adjacent normal mucosa. As a result, the field often is obscured by blood, thereby increasing the potential to damage important structures such as the middle turbinate, lamina papyracea, and cribriform plate. For these reasons, it has not been uncommon for the surgeon to abort the procedure before all the polyps have been removed. These patients have almost invariably required nasal packing for at least 24 hours. The soft-tissue shaver helps make the procedure routine. The shaver allows for excellent visualization of the anatomy while the polyps are precisely and quickly removed. Because the oscillating blade is guarded, important structures are less likely to be damaged. The continuous suction allows relatively uninterrupted dissection in a clear field. Packing is usually not required. Overall, a more complete removal is possible with less bleeding and greater comfort.

Postoperative Period

FESS is usually performed on an ambulatory basis. Most endoscopic sinus surgeons do not use any nasal packing after FESS. Patients seem to be much more comfortable when no packing is used. The postoperative care is as important as the surgery itself. Patients are instructed to use both saline nasal spray and saline irrigations in the nose several times a day to cleanse the nose of crusts and clots. This maintains a healthy, moist environment that will heal well. Weekly endoscopic cleanings are performed as necessary to prevent formation of granulation tissue, adhesions, and scars that can reobstruct drainage of the sinuses. Antibiotics and nasal corticosteroids are prescribed in the postoperative period. Antihistamines for allergic patients should be used with caution because they can lead to dryness, crusts, and thickened secretions. Usually the nasal mucosa has healed and normal mucociliary flow is reestablished within 6 weeks. Patients who undergo FESS for extensive sinonasal polyps require continued surveillance for months to years. The sinuses of post-FESS patients are easily accessible with office nasal endoscopy. Early regrowth of polyps can be identified and controlled by removing the polyps endoscopically in the office setting.

Complications of FESS

Complications of FESS include the same potential complications of traditional sinus surgeries. These include hemorrhage, scarring and formation of synechiae, injury to the orbit, and intracranial injury. Postoperative hemorrhage is uncommon with FESS, but is more likely in concomitant inferior turbinate resection or posterior middle turbinectomy. Scars or synechiae can form postoperatively and, if not recognized, can lead to sinus ostia obstruction and resurgence of sinus symptoms. Meticulous postoperative care by both the patient and otolaryngologist will prevent problems with synechiae. Orbital injuries may include exposure of orbital fat, hemorrhage into the orbit, extraocular muscle injury, globe injury, or optic nerve injury. Intracranial injuries may include cerebrospinal fluid leak, brain injury, or intracranial hemorrhage. Orbital and intracranial injuries are rare; however, the endoscopic surgeon must pay meticulous attention to surgical anatomic landmarks to avoid such possible complications.

Computer-Assisted Endoscopic Sinus Surgery (Image-Guided)

Computer-assisted surgery was initially developed for accurate localization during neurosurgical procedures. The application of this technique in endoscopic sinus surgery is in its early phases. Computer-assisted endoscopic sinus surgery can potentially aid the surgeon, especially when working in or near difficult areas such as the frontal sinuses, sphenoid sinus, skull base, and orbit. Computer-assisted endoscopic sinus surgery is still in its infancy. As it develops and becomes more available, its applications and advantages will require further evaluation.

Suggested Readings

Anon JB, Klimek L, Mosges R, et al: Computer-assisted endoscopic sinus surgery. An international review. *Otolaryngol Clin North Am* 1997;30:389-401.

Becker DG: Technical considerations in powered instrumentation. *Otolaryngol Clin North Am* 1997;30:421-434.

Dana ST: Out of committee. *Bull Am Acad Otolaryngol Head Neck Surg* 1994;13:12-14.

Fried MP: Intraoperative computerized imaging for endoscopic sinus surgery. *Vanderbilt University Sinus Newsletter*, Spring 1997.

Gross WE: Soft-tissue shavers in functional endoscopic sinus surgery (standard technique). *Otolaryngol Clin North Am* 1997;30:435-441.

Gross CW, Becker DG, eds. Advances in sinus and nasal surgery. *Otolaryngol Clin North Am* 1997;30:313-490.

Gustafson RO, Bansberg SF: Sinus surgery. In: Bailey BJ, ed. *Head and Neck Surgery—Otolaryngology*. Philadelphia, JB Lippincott, 1993, pp 377-388.

Kaliner MA, Osguthorpe JD, Fireman P, et al: Sinusitis: bench to bedside. Current findings, future directions. *Otolaryngol Head Neck Surg* 1997;116:S1-S20.

Kennedy DW, Senior BA: Endoscopic sinus surgery. A review. *Otolaryngol Clin North Am* 1997;30:313-330.

Lanza CL, Kennedy DW: Endoscopic sinus surgery. In: Bailey BJ, ed. *Head and Neck Surgery—Otolaryngology*. Philadelphia, JB Lippincott, 1993, pp 389-401.

Rice DH: Endoscopic sinus surgery. *Otolaryngol Clin North Am* 1993;26:613-618.

Setliff RC, Parsons DS: The "hummer": new instrumentation for functional endoscopic sinus surgery. *Am J Rhinol* 1994;8:275-278.

Stankiewicz JA: Complications of sinus surgery. In: Bailey BJ, ed. *Head and Neck Surgery—Otolaryngology*. Philadelphia, JB Lippincott, 1993, pp 413-427.

Chapter 11

The Pediatric Patient

The diagnosis of chronic sinusitis and frequent recurrent acute sinusitis in children remains somewhat controversial, especially in younger children, whose clinical presentation may be confusing and in whom abnormal radiographic findings may occur without sinusitis being present.

Diagnosis and Medical Management

The diagnosis should be based on clinical history and findings on physical examination, plus or minus laboratory results and imaging studies. Younger children will have less obvious clinical presentations; older children and adolescents present in the more obvious adult manner. The most common symptoms reported in young children are rhinorrhea (anterior or posterior), otitis media, cough, and irritability. Fetid breath also can occur. Persistent headache, facial pain, and fever are less common than in adults. A frequently overlooked subtle finding is mild periorbital edema, which is often present when the child awakens in the morning. Figure 1 outlines the development of the frontal and maxillary sinuses in children.

Sinusitis is an inflammation of the mucosal linings of the nose and paranasal sinuses. Active bacteriologic or viral infection need not be present. Sinusitis, particularly in the pediatric age group, generally accompanies or follows an up-

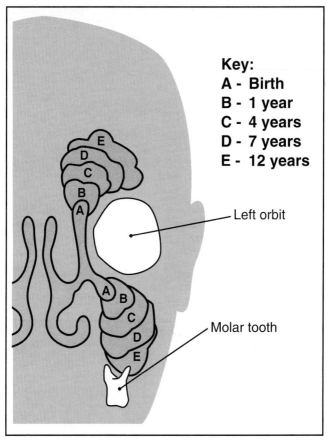

Figure 1: Pediatric development of the frontal and maxillary sinuses.

per respiratory infection, and may be secondary to or persist because of respiratory allergies or other systemic abnormalities or anatomic deformities.

Inflammatory disease of the paranasal sinuses most often responds to medical therapy, which is individualized for each patient depending on several factors. Most commonly, medical therapy includes antibiotics and a combination of decongestant preparations, humidifying medications, and anti-inflammatory nasal sprays. The medical regimen is similar to that described for adults in Chapter 9. Antihistamines or immunotherapy may be required in the allergic patient. Immunoglobulin therapy may be necessary in the child with immune deficiency. Patients with cystic fibrosis and sinusitis require aggressive comprehensive management by a cystic fibrosis specialist, as well as appropriate medical management for sinonasal polyposis and sinusitis. Pediatric patients with persistent sinusitis despite proper antibiotic, decongestant, nasal corticosteroid, and mucolytic therapy should be referred to an otolaryngologist and considered for allergic work-up, immunoglobulin levels including IgG subclasses, sweat chloride to rule out cystic fibrosis, and possible turbinate biopsy to rule out ciliary dyskinesia. Any child with nasal polyps should be suspected of having cystic fibrosis and, therefore, a sweat chloride test is required. In a small percentage of patients, sinusitis will fail to respond to even the most appropriate medical therapy. These children challenge even the most skilled practitioner, and may require surgical intervention to improve or cure their sinus disease.

Three primary conditions are necessary for the sinuses to function normally: (1) patent ostia; (2) normal mucociliary function; and (3) normal quality and quantity of secretions. Impairment of any one or a combination of these three components can lead to sinonasal inflammatory disease.

Conditions that may contribute to obstruction of the ostia are divided into two classes: mechanical and systemic. Mechanical obstruction can result from nasal tumors, polyps, synechiae, deviated nasal septum, hypertrophy of the turbinates, and inflammatory edema of the nasal and sinus mucosa. The latter is the most common cause of obstruction and is usually secondary to either upper respiratory tract infection or respiratory allergic disease. It has been estimated that patent ostia are present in only 20% of patients with acute rhinitis; therefore, sinusitis can easily develop in viral respiratory infections. Dysfunction of the normal mucociliary function, which commonly occurs after viral infections, is also seen in primary ciliary dyskinesia and leads to less effective clearance of secretions and subsequent ostium obstruction. Cystic fibrosis causes mucociliary dysfunction from hyperviscosity of the secretions, and these patients commonly experience obstructive polypoid disease. Upper respiratory infections and allergic inflammatory disease are the most common causes of chronic ostium obstruction. Allergic inflammatory disease causes nasal congestion through IgE-mediated release of histamine in the nasal mucosal membranes, resulting in mucosal edema and increased production of secretions in the sinus cavity, contributing to bacterial overgrowth. Many researchers have found a significant correlation between allergic disease and chronic sinusitis.

In the evaluation of a child with chronic or frequently recurring sinusitis, the presence of systemic disorders such as cystic fibrosis, immune disorder, primary ciliary dyskinesia including immotile cilia syndrome, and cyanotic heart disease must be considered. Proper management of these systemic conditions may obviate the need for intensive medical or surgical intervention for sinus disease. In patients with respiratory allergies and asthma who have sinusitis, these conditions may be brought under better control with continued aggressive medical management of both conditions. If this fails, surgical treatment may need to be added to the total management concept. When seizure disorders and sinusitis coexist, proper management of sinusitis frequently raises the seizure threshold. This may allow for seizure control with lower doses of anticonvulsants.

In the evaluation of potential surgical candidates, all pediatric patients should undergo a coronal computed tomographic (CT) scan of the sinuses. The techniques and principles are similar to those for adults. In children, individual modifications of surgery must be made according to the development of the paranasal sinuses and site of the anatomic structures. Therefore, it is even more important in children that CT scans provide detailed definition of structures and be of excellent quality, because small variations from the normal are critical. The cut of the CT scans is usually 3 to 4 mm. The procedure may require sedation and generally takes approximately 30 minutes to perform. General anesthesia is seldom necessary except in infants, but is recommended if needed to obtain adequate studies. The new spiral CT scans are much more efficient and require markedly less scanning time. Spiral CT offers the advantage of requiring little or no sedation in children because the scan is obtained much more rapidly. A bone algorithm is used to visualize the bony detail. In potential candidates for surgical intervention, we recommend obtaining the CT scan only after 4 weeks of intensive medical therapy. Patients who at that time demonstrate significant persistent disease and otherwise meet diagnostic criteria are considered possible surgical candidates. Findings on CT scan usually underestimate the pathologic conditions found in the operating room. Consequently, if other aspects of the diagnostic evaluation are sufficient to establish a diagnosis of sinusitis, a normal CT scan is not an absolute contraindication to surgery.

An additional feature that adds to the diagnostic problem is the difficulty of performing nasal endoscopy in children. This should not be used as an excuse not to attempt endoscopy. Young children often may be surprisingly cooperative with a gentle, patient approach. However, young children frequently require heavy sedation, or even general anesthesia, in addition to topical anesthesia and decongestants, before endoscopy can be completed. For these reasons, preoperative endoscopy need not always precede sinus surgery in children if all other criteria for surgery are met.

Functional Endoscopic Sinus Surgery (FESS) in Children

Functional endoscopic sinus surgery (FESS) in children is rapidly becoming the most accepted approach for children who require surgical intervention for chronic sinusitis and recurrent acute sinusitis. Approaches using nasal endoscopy are becoming mainstay surgical treatments for complications of

> **Table 1: Indications for FESS in Children Under 12 Years Old With Recurrent Acute Sinusitis**
>
> - 3 or fewer episodes of acute sinusitis in a child under 12 years of age: surgery *not* recommended
>
> - 4 or more episodes and no anatomic variant or a variant not causing ostiomeatal obstruction: surgery generally *not* advised unless the child has had an adenoidectomy, and immunotherapy if allergic
>
> - 4 or more episodes and evidence of ostiomeatal obstruction: surgery *may* be advised, especially for those who have had an adenoidectomy, and immunotherapy if allergic

sinusitis and for the management of other nasal and sinus conditions in children as well as adults.

Surgical intervention is reserved for those children in whom maximal prolonged medical therapy has failed. In such cases, we feel that surgical intervention is a more conservative approach than one that permits a child to become chronically ill (eg, develop chronic bronchitis) or to undergo unduly long and repeated courses of medical management. The final goals of any treatment regimen for sinusitis in children are to return the sinuses to as near a normal anatomic state as possible; to promote resolution of mucosal hypertrophy and infection; and thereby create a nasal-sinus environment that permits the sinuses to return to a normal disease-free state and development. Radical procedures to remove extensive amounts of mucous membranes from the sinuses are rarely indicated in children, even in patients with cystic fibrosis or other exacerbating conditions. Table 1 outlines indications for FESS in pediatric patients with recurrent acute sinusitis.

Complete resolution of acute sinusitis is the usual and expected outcome of any episode of sinusitis. Patients in whom

Table 2: Indications for FESS in Children Under 12 Years Old With Chronic Sinusitis

- Positive CT scan required before considering surgery

- Antibiotic treatment for a minimum of 21-28 days strongly advised; patients with a weak history and minimally positive imaging should be treated for more than 28 days

- Allergic patients with a history suggestive of sinusitis only should be given a trial of immuno-therapy; when history and imaging are strong, completion of a trial of immunotherapy not required if the patient has had an adenoidectomy, received nasal corticosteroids, and has had more than 28 days of antibiotics

- Adenoidectomy generally advised before sinus surgery

- Use of oral or topical corticosteroids may be effective for sinusitis in children and should be used if potential benefit outweighs risk

more conservative therapy has failed (including maximal medical therapy, adenoidectomy or adenotonsillectomy, and allergy therapy), and who continue to have frequent recurrent episodes of sinusitis or symptoms of chronic sinusitis, are potential candidates for FESS.

Recurrent episodes of acute sinusitis in children under 12 years of age are almost always treated medically using antibiotics, decongestants, and nasal corticosteroids. Immunotherapy should be strongly considered in the allergic child. Adenoidectomy is generally recommended before considering sinus surgery. The surgical option is not recommended for fewer than 4 recurrences of acute sinusitis.

Surgery for chronic sinusitis in children may be indicated when: medical management fails; allergy either has been ruled out or a trial of immunotherapy has been unsuccessful; adenoids have been removed; and a CT scan is positive for sinus disease. Medical management includes antibiotics for at least 21 to 28 days in addition to nasal corticosteroids and decongestants. Table 2 outlines indications for FESS in pediatric patients with chronic sinusitis.

Pediatric FESS Technique

The technique for FESS in children is essentially the same as described for adults in the last chapter. The operating field is smaller in children and, with each patient, individual consideration must be given to the site and extent of development of the sinuses, as well as the extent of the disease as shown on the CT scan. For this reason, the CT scan is frequently referred to throughout the procedure. The sinus instruments have been modified for use in the more constricted pediatric anatomy. Smaller-diameter 2.7-mm nasal endoscopes are available for use in children with narrow nasal cavities and sinus spaces. However, for most pediatric FESS cases, we are able to use the adult 4.0-mm nasal endoscopes. The 4-mm endoscope is preferred over the smaller endoscope because illumination is far better, the field of vision is much broader, and we seem to have better depth perception than with the smaller endoscope.

Postoperative Period After Pediatric FESS

Oral antibiotics, topical nasal decongestants, topical nasal corticosteroid spray, and saline nasal spray are administered postoperatively. The saline spray is used frequently and copiously to prevent drying and crusting in the nasal cavity. Adolescents, like adults, will be able to cooperate with essential endoscopic weekly postoperative cleaning of clots and granulation. Younger children, however, cannot tolerate the endoscopic cleaning in the office. Therefore, for optimal results, the younger child returns to the operating room at 2 weeks for second-stage cleaning to divide synechiae, remove clots and excess granulation tissue, and irrigate the maxillary sinuses through the maxillary antrostomy. Postoperative medications are gradually discontinued on an individual basis. Some patients require chronic use of topical nasal corticosteroids.

Results of Pediatric FESS

We have obtained good results with FESS in children in more than 80% of cases with no serious complications (eg, orbital or intracranial complications). Seven percent have required revision surgery. We feel that FESS is the method of choice in the child who is severely affected by sinusitis and does not respond to the most thorough and appropriate medical regimen. This surgery does require special training, and should be done only by those experienced in endoscopic sinus surgery.

Suggested Readings

Dana ST: Out of committee. *Bull Am Acad Otolaryngol Head Neck Surg* 1994;13:12-14.

Gross CW, Avner TG, Becker DG: Sinusitis in children. In: Gates GA, ed. *Current Therapy in Otolaryngology—Head and Neck Surgery*, 5th ed. St. Louis, Mosby-Year Book, 1994, pp 373-377.

Gross CW, Lazar RH, Gurucharri MJ: Pediatric functional endonasal sinus surgery. *Otolaryngol Clin North Am* 1989;22:733-738.

Gross CW, Gurucharri MJ, Lazar RH, et al: Functional endonasal sinus surgery (FESS) in the pediatric age group. *Laryngoscope* 1989;99:272-275.

Lazar RH, Younis RT, Long TE: Functional endonasal sinus surgery in adults and children. *Laryngoscope* 1993;103:1-5.

Lusk RP: *Pediatric Sinusitis*. New York, Raven Press, 1992.

Manning SC: Pediatric sinusitis. *Otolaryngol Clin North Am* 1993;26:623-638.

Chapter 12

Complications and Emergencies Associated With Sinusitis

The orbit and intracranial structures are close to the paranasal sinuses. As a result, sinus infections potentially lead to orbital or intracranial complications. Therefore, the risk of morbidity and even mortality is significant.

Orbital Complications of Sinusitis

The orbit is adjacent to the ethmoid sinuses, separated only by the paper-thin lamina papyracea. Infections in the ethmoid sinuses can spread directly to the orbit either by penetration of the lamina papyracea or through small dehiscences in the bone. Such dehiscences often are congenital, but may also be produced by previous surgery or trauma. Direct extension of infection can also occur through the anterior and posterior ethmoid foramina, through which the anterior and posterior ethmoid vessels pass from the orbit through the medial orbital wall to the ethmoid sinuses. Thrombophlebitis can spread through these vessels to the orbit. The ophthalmic venous system represents another potential source for spread of infection. This venous system lacks valves, allowing easier communication among the face, nasal cavity, paranasal sinuses, orbits, and cavernous sinus.

Classification

Chandler provided a classification system for evaluation of orbital infection secondary to sinusitis. These range from

Table 1: Classification of Orbital Complications of Sinusitis

Class 1: Inflammatory eyelid edema or preseptal cellulitis

Class 2: Orbital cellulitis

Class 3: Subperiosteal abscess

Class 4: Orbital abscess

Class 5: Cavernous sinus thrombosis

class 1 to class 5 as the severity of orbital infection increases (Table 1). This classification system is helpful for making accurate diagnoses and guiding management.

Inflammatory eyelid edema or preseptal cellulitis (class 1) is the most common of the five classes. Patients with this condition present with typical signs and symptoms of sinusitis associated with edema and erythema of the eyelid. These eyelid findings are attributable to venous obstruction caused by pressure on the ethmoid vessels by the infection. The eyelid swelling can become quite impressive. The eyelid may even become swollen shut, but with no associated proptosis, limitation of extraocular muscle motility, or visual impairment. This condition is often referred to as *preseptal cellulitis* because the infection remains anterior to the orbital septum in the eyelid. The tarsal plate and orbital septum act as barriers to limit the infection to the eyelid and prevent spread to the orbital contents.

Orbital cellulitis (class 2) represents inflammation and cellulitis of the orbital contents. The orbit is involved, with diffuse edema and inflammatory and bacterial infiltration of adipose tissue. There is no abscess formation. This results in proptosis (anterior protrusion of the globe) and chemosis (inflammatory edema of the bulbar conjunctiva). Extraocular muscle motility may be limited because of muscle edema and spasm. Vision may be impaired, depending on severity.

Subperiosteal abscess (class 3) represents a circumscribed collection of pus at the medial orbit between the bone and the periorbita. The periorbita acts as a barrier to spread of the infection. The abscess in this location can cause lateral and downward displacement of the globe. Orbital cellulitis is often simultaneously present, causing impairment of extraocular muscle motility because of muscle edema and spasm. In the early stages, vision is normal, but may become impaired as the severity of the orbital infection increases.

Orbital abscess (class 4) represents pus formation in the orbital soft tissues behind the globe. It is thought to develop secondary to extension of infection into orbital fat with inflammatory edema, fat necrosis, and frank pus formation. This causes marked proptosis, chemosis, and severe limitation of extraocular muscle motility. Vision is usually impaired. This may be attributable to increased orbital pressure with retinal artery occlusion or optic neuritis. Permanent blindness may result if prompt surgical and medical therapy is not expeditiously employed.

Cavernous sinus thrombosis (class 5) results from spread of orbital infection to the cavernous sinus. Such spread is attributable to the lack of valves in the orbital veins that communicate with the cavernous sinus. The important clinical signs are orbital pain, proptosis, rapidly progressive chemosis and limitation of extraocular muscle motility, marked retinal venous engorgement, spread of orbital cellulitis to the opposite eye, and clinical deterioration of the patient with sepsis. Meningitis is often present. Blindness and death may result.

Diagnosis

The diagnosis of orbital involvement in sinusitis is made by history, physical examination, laboratory evaluation, and radiographic studies. The history usually reveals a recent upper respiratory infection with or without nasal discharge. Pain over the involved sinuses may be present. Orbital signs on physical examination are lid edema, chemosis, proptosis, limitation of extraocular muscle motility, and visual loss. Ophthalmologic examination is essential to assess the status of the eye and to exclude concurrent ocular problems. Nasal examination may reveal discharge near the middle meatus. Laboratory tests should include a complete blood count (CBC), differential, sedimentation rate, and blood cultures. Plain x-rays of the sinuses can be valuable by showing opacification or an air-fluid level within the involved sinus. However, computed tomography (CT) scan is better and is the recommended imaging study for evaluation of orbital complications of sinusitis. Soft-tissue abnormalities with orbital cellulitis and abscess are well demonstrated on CT. When the clinician suspects orbital infection from sinusitis, the CT scan should be performed with intravenous contrast to help clarify and delineate the presence of abscess formation. Certainly, the CT scan helps determine the class of the orbital infection and guide the management.

Microbiology and Antibiotic Therapy

Studies show that more than 50% of cases of acute sinusitis, regardless of severity, are caused by *Streptococcus pneumoniae* and *Haemophilus influenzae*. *Moraxella catarrhalis* and *Staphylococcus aureus* are important but contribute less frequently. Antibiotics are chosen to encompass these microorganisms. The choice of agents depends on many factors, including in vitro susceptibility of bacteria in the specific geographic area, and comorbid disease (see Chapter 8). Severely ill patients with sinusitis should be evaluated by an infectious disease specialist.

Treatment

The treatment of orbital complications of sinusitis depends on the severity of the signs and symptoms. However, even the earlier stages must be treated aggressively to prevent progression. Patients with inflammatory eyelid edema or preseptal cellulitis (class 1) can be treated with oral antibiotics in certain cases if the edema is mild and the patient has not received prior treatment. However, attentive close follow-up is required, and the treating physician should have a low threshold for admitting the patient for IV antibiotics and close ob-

Table 2: Medical Therapy for Sinusitis With Orbital Complication

- Antibiotics
- Systemic decongestants
- Topical decongestants
- Head of bed elevation
- Warm compresses
- Saline nasal drops or spray
- Humidification
- Hydration
- Analgesics

servation. All patients with evidence of postseptal involvement (classes 2-5) should be hospitalized for IV antibiotics and close observation. In patients with orbital cellulitis (class 2, postseptal involvement with no abscess formation), the initial treatment is medical.

In addition to the antibiotics, the medical regimen consists of both systemic and topical decongestants, elevation of the head of the bed, warm compresses, humidification, intravenous fluids, and analgesics (Table 2). Close monitoring of visual acuity and extraocular muscle motility is essential. Resolution or progression is assessed by clinical examination, including visual acuity, extraocular muscle motility, temperature, and white blood cell (WBC) count, as well as by sequential CT scan imaging. Outcome of medical management depends on duration and stage of orbital involvement.

Surgical intervention is generally indicated in patients with any CT scan evidence of abscess formation, deterioration of visual acuity, signs of progressive orbital involvement despite adequate medical therapy, lack of response to adequate medical therapy, relapse, or any evidence of involvement of the opposite eye (Table 3). Surgery is aimed at drain-

Table 3: Indications for Surgery

- Abscess formation on CT scan
- Deterioration of visual acuity
- Progression despite adequate medical therapy
- Lack of response to adequate medical therapy
- Relapse
- Involvement of the opposite eye

ing any abscess formation and allowing proper drainage of the involved sinus.

The most common surgical procedure is an external ethmoidectomy, which starts with a curvilinear incision between the medial canthus of the eye and the midline of the nose. A subperiosteal abscess is drained along the medial orbit via this approach. If an orbital abscess is present, an incision is made into the periorbita between the superior and medial rectus muscles. Ethmoidectomy for the involved ethmoid sinus usually is performed by this approach, and communication is created intranasally to the middle meatus. A drain is left in the cavity and brought into the middle meatus after completion of the external ethmoidectomy. If CT scan evidence suggests frontal sinus opacification, trephination of the frontal sinus can be performed through the same incision, and an irrigation tube can be inserted if an abscess is found. If maxillary sinusitis is present, an antrostomy and irrigation is done. Appropriate medical therapy as described is continued in the postoperative period.

Alternatively, many endoscopic surgeons have recently supported an endoscopic approach for treatment of subperiosteal abscess (class 3). This involves intranasal endoscopic ethmoidectomy and drainage of the subperiosteal abscess without the need for an external incision. Orbital abscess (class 4) is still approached with an external incision.

Complete return of visual acuity should occur within a few days following surgical drainage of the orbit and involved sinuses. If improvement in the patient's general condition and visual acuity is not prompt, a persistent orbital abscess should be suspected. Even when visual acuity improves relatively quickly, the proptosis, periorbital induration, and extraocular muscle motility return more gradually. Complete resolution can take as long as 2 to 3 months.

Mucocele

Chronic sinusitis can lead to the formation of a primary or secondary mucocele. Primary mucoceles are mucus retention cysts. Secondary mucoceles are those caused by inflammation and scarring of the sinus ostia as a result of chronic sinusitis or trauma. Mucoceles are epithelial-lined cavities containing fluid. The epithelium of the mucocele is low columnar or cuboidal, while normal sinus epithelium is ciliated, columnar respiratory epithelium. Mucoceles are most common in the frontal sinus. Ethmoid, maxillary, and sphenoid mucoceles are less common, and have the potential to slowly invade and apply chronic pressure on surrounding vital structures such as the orbit and brain. A mucocele that becomes infected and contains pus is a *mucopyocele*. A mucopyocele that ruptures intracranially can be dangerous.

Mucoceles are best evaluated with CT scan to delineate details of bony invasion. Magnetic resonance imaging (MRI) can provide the soft-tissue detail needed to rule out tumor. Frontal mucoceles are treated by excision with obliteration or ablation of the sinus. Ethmoid, maxillary, and sphenoid mucoceles are usually treated with marsupialization, either via traditional approaches or endoscopically.

Osteomyelitis

Sinusitis can lead to osteomyelitis, or bone infection. This occurs either by direct extension of infection or by thrombophlebitic involvement of the diploic veins. Osteomyelitis of the frontal sinus can lead to subperiosteal abscess of the frontal bone. This presents as a doughy swelling of the forehead known as *Pott's puffy tumor*. Osteomyelitis of the maxilla and sphenoid bone is much less common. The microorganism

Table 4: Intracranial Complications of Sinusitis

- Meningitis
- Epidural abscess
- Subdural abscess
- Venous sinus thrombosis
- Brain abscess

usually involved is *S aureus*. The treatment consists of surgical drainage and appropriate antibiotics. Débridement of infected bone is rarely necessary when long-term intravenous antibiotics are employed.

Intracranial Complications of Sinusitis

Intracranial complications of sinusitis are rare, especially in the antibiotic era. These potentially life-threatening complications include meningitis, epidural abscess, subdural abscess, venous sinus thrombosis, and brain abscess (Table 4). The physician who treats patients with sinusitis must keep these potential complications in mind. It is important to recognize neurologic signs and obtain the appropriate otolaryngologic, infectious disease, neurologic, and neurosurgical consultations when such complications are recognized.

Suggested Readings

Arjmand EM, Lusk RP, Muntz HR: Pediatric sinusitis and subperiosteal orbital abscess formation: diagnosis and treatment. *Otolaryngol Head Neck Surg* 1993;109:886-894.

Chandler JR, Langenbrunner DJ, Stevens ER: The pathogenesis of orbital complications in acute sinusitis. *Laryngoscope* 1970;80:1414-1428.

Clayman GL, Adams GL, Paugh DR, et al: Intracranial complications of paranasal sinusitis: a combined institutional review. *Laryngoscope* 1991;101:234-239.

Fairbanks DNF, Vanderveen TS, Bradley JE: Intracranial complications of sinusitis. In: English GM, ed. *Otolaryngology*, vol 2. Philadelphia, Harper and Row, 1987.

Manning SC: Endoscopic management of medial subperiosteal orbital abscess. *Arch Otolaryngol Head Neck Surg* 1993;119:789-791.

Osguthorpe JD, Hochman M: Inflammatory sinus diseases affecting the orbit. *Otolaryngol Clin North Am* 1993;26:657-671.

Stankiewicz JA, Newell DJ, Park AH: Complications of inflammatory diseases of the sinuses. *Otolaryngol Clin North Am* 1993;26:639-655.

Chapter 13

Quality of Life

Traditionally, outcome analysis of medical care has focused on assessment of morbidity. More recently, outcome analysis has begun to focus more on assessment of the patient's health-related quality of life (HRQL). HRQL information comes directly from the patients, and relates to their sense of well-being and ability to perform day-to-day activities in relation to their illness.

To analyze quality of life, questionnaires have been developed to produce reliable, valid, and reproducible data. HRQL measures usually include: (1) a general health assessment, and (2) a disease-specific assessment. Quality-of-life measures may be obtained with respect to a specific disease, before or after specific treatments.

The most common general health assessment survey is the Medical Outcomes Study Short Form 36-Item Health Survey (SF-36). This survey focuses on eight subscales of general health, including physical functioning, role functioning, bodily pain, general health, level of energy, social functioning, emotional functioning, and mental health (Table 1). In a study using SF-36, patients with chronic sinusitis were found to have significant decreases in quality-of-life measures compared with normal levels. The subscales that were most affected were role functioning, bodily pain, general health, level of energy, and social functioning. Such decrements in

Table 1: Eight Subscales of General Health: The SF-36 Survey

Subscale	Parameters
PF	Limitation on physical activities such as walking, bathing, and strenuous sports
RP	Problems with work or other daily activities because of physical health
BP	Intensity of bodily pain or limitations because of pain
GH	Perception of current health and health outlook
VT	Level of energy
SF	Extent to which health interferes with normal social activities
RE	Problems with daily activities resulting from emotional issues
MH	Mental health screening

quality of life for chronic sinusitis patients were similar to those seen in other chronic diseases such as chronic obstructive pulmonary disease, congestive heart failure, and angina pectoris.

The most common disease-specific assessment for chronic sinusitis is the Chronic Sinusitis Survey (CSS) (Table 2). This survey contains six disease-related questions: three related to duration of symptoms, and three related to duration of medication use. The symptoms assessed are: (1) sinus headaches, facial pain, or pressure; (2) nasal drainage or postnasal drip; and (3) nasal congestion or obstruction. The medications assessed are: (1) antibiotics; (2) prescription nasal sprays; and (3) oral sinus medications such as decongestants and antihistamines.

Gliklich and Metson reported on the effect of sinus surgery on quality of life in 1997. This study used SF-36 for general health assessment and CSS for disease-specific assessment.

Table 2: Chronic Sinusitis Survey (CSS)

Name_____

Date_____

This survey asks for your view about your sinus symptoms and treatment. This information will remain in your medical record to help your doctor keep track of how you feel.

Answer every question by circling the appropriate number. If you are unsure about how to answer a question, please give the best answer you can.

1. During the past **8 weeks,** how many **weeks** have you had: (circle one answer in each row)
   a. Sinus headaches, facial pain, or pressure
          0   1-2   3-4   5-6   7-8
   b. Nasal drainage or postnasal drip
          0   1-2   3-4   5-6   7-8
   c. Nasal congestion or difficulty breathing through your nose
          0   1-2   3-4   5-6   7-8

2. During the past **8 weeks,** how many **weeks** have you taken: (circle one answer in each row)
   a. Antibiotics
          0   1-2   3-4   5-6   7-8
   b. Nasal sprays prescribed by your doctor
          0   1-2   3-4   5-6   7-8
   c. Sinus medications in pill form (such as antihistamines, decongestants)
          0   1-2   3-4   5-6   7-8

3. Who completed this form? (Circle one number)
   a. I filled it out myself   1
   b. Someone asked me the questions   2
   c. By telephone   3

4. Have you had any revision surgery in the past year on your sinuses? (for 1-year postsurgery patients only)
            Yes   No

The surveys were completed by 160 patients. Of these, 108 patients underwent endoscopic sinus surgery and completed surveys at a minimum of 6 months postoperatively. The remaining 52 patients were treated with medical therapy alone and completed surveys through a 3-month period.

In this study, 82% of patients who underwent surgery for chronic sinusitis demonstrated statistically significant clinical improvement in their sinusitis-specific measures on CSS. Patients who underwent surgery for chronic sinusitis demonstrated significant improvement on SF-36 in six of the eight subscales of general health 12 months after surgery. Patients with coexisting asthma began the study with lower general health scores, but demonstrated significant improvements after sinus surgery, reaching levels similar to those of the nonasthma patients who underwent surgery. Patients who received medical therapy only demonstrated significant improvements in sinusitis-specific scores, but not to the same degree as patients who underwent surgery. This comparison of the surgical group and the nonsurgical group is not substantiated, however, because this study did not randomize these groups. The methods used in this study, however, seem suitable for future studies comparing surgical and medical modalities for chronic sinusitis.

Health-related quality-of-life measures represent the newest method of outcome assessment. Poor quality of life, severity of symptoms, and prolonged medication use lead the patient to pursue surgical intervention for chronic sinusitis. As a result, HRQL measures are greatly applicable to the study of chronic sinusitis and its treatment. We will certainly see multiple quality-of-life studies on sinusitis soon. Results of these studies may improve the ability of health-care providers to inform their patients of the outcomes of the available treatments.

Suggested Readings

Bowen OR: Shattuck lecture—what is quality care? *N Engl J Med* 1987;316:1578-1580.

Gliklich RE, Hilinski JM: Longitudinal sensitivity of generic and specific health measures in chronic sinusitis. *Qual Life Res* 1995;4:27-32.

Gliklich RE, Metson R: The health impact of chronic sinusitis in patients seeking otolaryngologic care. *Otolaryngol Head Neck Surg* 1995;113:104-109.

Gliklich RE, Metson R: Techniques for outcomes research in chronic sinusitis. *Laryngoscope* 1995;105:387-390.

Gliklich RE, Metson R: Effect of sinus surgery on quality of life. *Otolaryngol Head Neck Surg* 1997;117:12-17.

Hoffman SR, Mahoney MC, Chmiel JF, et al: Symptom relief after endoscopic sinus surgery: an outcomes-based study. *Ear Nose Throat J* 1993;72:413-414.

Kaliner MA, Osguthorpe JD, Fireman P, et al: Sinusitis: bench to bedside. Current findings, future directions. *Otolaryngol Head Neck Surg* 1997;116:S1-S20.

Ware JE Jr, Sherbourne CD: The MOS 36-item short-form health survey (SF-36). I. Conceptual framework and item selection. *Med Care* 1992;30:473-483.

Ware JE, ed: *The SF-36 health survey manual and interpretation guide*. Boston, Nimrod Press, 1993.

Index

A

abscess   130

Absidia   77

acquired immune deficiency syndrome (AIDS)   26, 30, 36, 41, 74, 78

adenoid hypertrophy   41

adenoidectomy   121, 122

adenotonsillectomy   122

adhesions   113

Aerobid®   95

Aerospace Medical Association   10

Afrin®   92

agger nasi   14, 17

air pollutants   9

air travel   10

alcohol   9

Allegra™   99

allergens   9, 26, 99

allergies   91, 97, 101, 103, 117

allergy   10, 37, 75, 109

allergy testing   46

allergy therapy   122

Alternaria   74

amoxicillin   83, 84, 88, 94

amoxicillin/clavulanate (Augmentin®)   28, 81, 82, 84-88, 90

amphotericin B (Fungizone®)   76, 77

ampicillin   83, 84, 88

anaphylaxis   88

anesthesia   43

anticonvulsants   119

antidepressants   102

antihistamines   5, 8, 10, 38, 46, 65, 79, 92-95, 97-99, 101-103, 113, 118, 135

antiretroviral therapy   79

Antivert®   99

antrostomy   109, 123, 130

aspergillosis   75, 77

Aspergillus   29, 30, 38, 74, 76, 78, 79, 89

Aspergillus flavus   75

Aspergillus fumigatus   75

Aspergillus niger   75

aspirin intolerance   91

astemizole (Hismanal®)   99

asthma   106, 119, 137

Atarax®   99

atomizers   10

atresia   107

Augmentin®   28, 81

azithromycin (Zithromax®)   82, 83, 85-88, 90

B

bacteria   30

Bacteroides   29

Bactrim™   83

barotrauma   36, 41

basal lamella   14, 18, 111

bathing   135

beclomethasone dipropionate (Vancenase®, Beconase®)   95

Beconase®   95, 96

Benadryl®   99

Biaxin®   28, 81

bicuspid teeth   15

biopsy   45

Bipolaris   76

birth control pills   25

black molds   74

bleeding   96

blindness   127

Bonine®   99

brain abscess   132

brain injury   114

bronchitis   11, 106, 121

bronchopneumonia   73, 74

bronchopulmonary aspergillosis   30

bronchopulmonary disease   75, 76

budesonide (Rhinocort®)   95

burning   96, 100

C

calcium   85

Candida   30, 74

canthus pain   37

cardiac pacemakers   57

CD4 levels   45

cefprozil (Cefzil®)   28, 81, 82, 84, 85, 86, 87

Ceftin®   28, 81

ceftriaxone (Rocephin®)   87, 88, 90

cefuroxime axetil (Ceftin®)   28, 81, 82, 84-87

Cefzil®   28, 81

cerebrospinal fluid leak   114

cetirizine (Zyrtec®)   99, 100

Charcot-Leyden crystals   30

chemosis   126, 127

chills   37

Chlamydia   88

Chlamydia pneumoniae   27, 28, 30

Chlor-Trimeton®   99

chloramphenicol (Chloromycetin®)   88, 90

Chloromycetin®   88

chlorpheniramine maleate (Chlor-Trimeton®)   99

choanal atresia   36, 41

Chronic Sinusitis Survey (CSS)   135-137

cigarette smoke   26

cigarette smoking   9, 78

cilia   19, 21, 23, 45, 107

ciliary dyskinesia   45, 118, 119

ciliary dysmotility   41

ciliated epithelium   49

Cipro®   28, 78, 81

ciprofloxacin (Cipro®)   28, 78, 81, 82, 84-86, 88

clarithromycin (Biaxin®)   28, 81, 82, 85-88, 90

Claritin®   99

Claritin®-D   100

Claritin®-D 24   100

claustrophobia   57

clindamycin   84

cocaine   78, 110

collagen vascular disease   41

columnar epithelium   17

common cold   26, 37, 57

complete blood count (CBC)   45, 128

computed tomography (CT)   5, 26, 37, 47, 51-66, 68, 73, 74, 76, 86, 106, 109, 111, 119, 120, 122, 123, 128-131

concha bullosa   25, 43, 55, 111

congestion   97

congestive heart failure   135

corticosteroids   10, 77, 79, 94, 98, 99, 101

Corynebacterium   29

cost-containment concerns   53

cough   37, 40, 76, 97, 116

cough syrups   97

cow's milk   102

cranial fossa   15

cribriform plate   14, 112

cromolyn   92

cromolyn sodium (Nasalcrom®)   98-101, 103

cromolyn spray   46

crusting   96, 98

crusts   113

Curvularia   76

cyanotic heart disease   119

cystic fibrosis   23, 30, 41, 45, 46, 49, 91, 118, 119, 121

cysts   131

Cytomegalovirus   79

D

dacryocystorhinostomy   107

dander   98

débridement   77, 132

decongestants   10, 38, 41, 43, 65, 79, 89, 91-96, 98-100, 103, 109, 118, 120, 122, 123, 129, 135

deviated nasal septum   9, 25, 36, 41, 111, 118

diabetes mellitus   26, 30, 74

diphenhydramine (Benadryl®)   99

diphtheria toxoid conjugate   45

Doryx®   83

dosimetry 68

doxycycline (Doryx®, Vibramycin®) 82-90

dryness 96, 98, 113

dust 46

dust mites 26, 98

E

edema 42, 86, 118, 119, 126, 127

electron microscopy 45

empyema 61, 73

endoscope 42

endoscopic evaluation 86

endoscopic sinus surgery 137

endoscopic surgery 11, 107

endoscopy 5, 8, 27, 42, 60, 109

Enterobacteriaceae 26

environmental controls 103

eosinophils 30

epidural abscess 132

epinephrine 110

epithelial cells 19

epithelium 12, 23, 107

erythema 41, 42, 86, 126

erythrocyte sedimentation rate (ESR or SED rate) 45

erythromycin 84

ethmoid bulla 18, 19, 21, 43, 110

ethmoid fluid cells 12

ethmoid foramina 125

ethmoidectomy 111, 130

eustachian tube obstruction 44

eyelid edema 126, 128

F

facial numbness 59

facial pain 37, 40, 58, 116, 135

facial pressure 40

fat necrosis 127

fatigue 40

fetal sinus development 9

fetid breath 116

fever 37, 40, 61, 72-74, 76, 78, 116

fexofenadine (Allegra™) 99, 100

Flonase™ 95

flunisolide (Aerobid®, Nasarel™) 95

fluoroquinolones 90

fluticasone (Flonase™) 95

food allergy 102, 103

Food and Drug Administration (FDA) 28, 81, 82

fovea ethmoidalis 14, 111

functional endoscopic sinus surgery (FESS) 43, 51-53, 63, 66, 106-110, 113, 120-124

fungal hyphae 30

fungal infections 30, 63

Fungizone® 76

Fusobacterium 29

G

General Health: The SF-36 Survey   135

GI discomfort   97

global warming   9

Gomori's methenamine silver (GMS) stain   76

granulocyte colony-stimulating factor (GCSF)   77

granulocytopenia   77

grasses   98

guaifenesin   79, 97

H

Haemophilus influenzae   9, 10, 27, 28, 30, 45, 78, 81, 82, 84, 88, 89, 92, 94, 128

halitosis   40

Haller air cell   55

head trauma   12

headache   37, 38, 40, 66, 76, 78, 116, 135

helium   69

hemochromatosis   77

hemodialysis   26, 28

hemorrhage   113, 114

hiatus semilunaris   18-20, 43

Hismanal®   99

histamine   5, 98, 100, 119

Horner's syndrome   91

house dust   26

human immunodeficiency virus (HIV)   45, 72, 78, 79

humidification   12, 13, 48, 92-95, 97, 129

hydration   129

hydroxyzine (Atarax®)   99

hyperbaric oxygenation   78

hypersensitivity reaction   103

hypertrophy   36, 118, 121

hypophysectomy   107

hypothyroidism   91

hypoxia   23, 107

I

IgA deficiency   41, 45

IgE   119

IgE antibodies   97, 102

IgE levels   78

IgG   45, 78, 118

IgG subtype deficiency   25

imaging   53

immotile cilia   91

immotile cilia syndrome   23, 45, 119

immune deficiency   41, 91

immunoglobulin   25

immunoglobulin deficiency   45

immunoglobulin therapy   118

immunosuppression therapy   30

immunotherapy   46, 92, 98, 99, 101-103, 109, 118, 121-123

infertility   45

inflammation   107, 131

influenza vaccine   10, 89

infraorbital ethmoid air cell   55

infundibulum   14, 16, 18-20

interferon   19

International Conference on
Sinus Disease   5

intersinus septa   15

intersinus septum   16

intracranial hemorrhage   114

intracranial infections   73

intracranial injury   113

intranasal cocaine   25

iron   85

irritability   116

irritation   96, 100

itching   98

itchy nose   46

itchy or watery eyes   46

itchy palate   46

itraconazole (Sporanox®)   30, 76

K

Kartagener's syndrome   23, 41

ketoacidosis   77

ketoconazole (Nizoral®)   99

L

lactoferrin   19

lamina papyracea   14, 18, 111,
112, 125

Legionella   27, 28, 88

leukemia   77

leukotrienes   100

Levaquin®   28, 82

levofloxacin (Levaquin®)   28,
82, 84-89

lidocaine   110

lidocaine (Xylocaine®)   43

longus colli   56

Lorabid®   28, 82

loracarbef (Lorabid®)   28, 82,
84-87

loratadine (Claritin®)   99, 100

lysozymes   19

M

magnesium   85

magnetic resonance (MR)   51,
53, 56, 60, 66, 68, 69

magnetic resonance imaging
(MRI)   26, 56, 63, 64, 131

malodorous breath   41

marsupialization   131

masseter   56

maxillary dental disease   84

maxillary dental sepsis   37

maxillary toothache   38, 58, 86

meatus   14, 15, 18, 23, 42-44,
107, 109, 110, 130

meclizine (Antivert®,
Bonine®)   99

Medical Outcomes Study
Short Form 36-Item
Health Survey   134

membrane   17

meningitis 38, 127, 132

mental changes 38

methicillin-resistant
  S aureus 30

Microsporidia 79

molars 15

molds 46, 98

Moraxella catarrhalis 27, 28,
  30, 78, 81, 82, 84, 88, 89, 94,
  128

mucocele 60, 131

mucociliary clearance 19, 23,
  45, 52

mucociliary dysfunction 25,
  109

mucolytics 92, 94, 95, 97, 109

mucopyocele 131

Mucor 29, 74, 77

mucormycosis 76, 77

mucosal edema 72

mucosal hypertrophy 41

mucus ciliary clearance 79

muscle injury 114

mycetoma 75, 76

*Mycobacterium avium-
  intracellulare* 79

Mycoplasma 88

Mycoplasma pneumoniae 27,
  28, 30

mycotic genera 74

N

Nasacort® 95

nasal congestion 10, 46, 119,
  135

nasal corticosteroid spray 101,
  123

nasal corticosteroids 93, 95,
  101, 103, 107, 109, 113, 118,
  122, 124

nasal discharge 37, 127

nasal drainage 135

nasal endoscopes 106, 110,
  111, 123

nasal endoscopy 47, 53, 61,
  67, 106, 120

nasal lavage 92-96

nasal obstruction 37, 40, 42,
  43

nasal polyps 11, 46, 100, 112

nasal saline 65, 96

nasal sprays 101, 118, 135

Nasalcrom® 46, 100

Nasarel™ 95, 96

National Center for Disease
  Statistics 7

nebulizers 10

neoplasm 60

Nizoral® 99

O

occipital pain 37

ocular dysfunction 60

ofloxacin   84

olfaction   12

olfactory disturbance   40

optic nerve injury   114

optic neuritis   127

oral candidiasis   30

orbital abscess   126, 127, 130, 131

orbital cellulitis   126, 127, 129

orbital infection   126-128

orbital pain   127

orbitopathy   107

osteomyelitis   131

ostia   5, 9, 37, 131

ostiomeatal complex (OMC)   5, 17, 18, 20, 23, 25, 40, 47, 55, 66, 72, 79, 86, 89, 91, 92, 94, 95, 106-109, 111
   OMC obstruction   23, 121

ostium   15, 18, 111

otitis media   38, 41, 116

otoscopy   73, 74

oxymetazoline (Afrin®)   41, 92, 110

P

pain   134, 135

pain in the cheeks   37

pain in the forehead   37

PBZ®   99

penicillin   87

penicillin-resistant
   S pneumoniae   30

perfume   26

periorbital edema   116

pet dander   46

phaeohyphomycosis   74, 76

Phenergan®   99

phenylephrine   42, 43, 110

phenylpropanolamine   96

phototoxicity   85

Phycomycetes   29, 74, 77

plain-film radiography   68

plain-film x-rays   58-60, 67, 73

pneumococcal disease   78

pneumococcal vaccine   10, 89

pneumonia   11, 74

pollens   98

polypoid disease   119

polyposis   62, 118

polyps   25, 36, 41-43, 59, 60, 91, 111, 113, 118

Pontocaine®   43

postnasal discharge   97

postnasal drainage   41

postnasal drip   40, 43, 98, 135

Pott's puffy tumor   131

pregnant women   9

preseptal cellulitis   126, 128

ProHIBiT®   45

promethazine (Phenergan®)   99

proptosis   60, 62, 126, 127, 131

prostaglandins   100

provocative food test (PFT)   103

pruritus   97

pseudoephedrine   92, 96, 100

Pseudomonas aeruginosa   73, 78, 89

pterygoid   56

pterygomaxillary fossae   15

puberty   25

pulmonary disease   135

purulent secretions   42, 44

pyocele   60

Q

quality of life   134, 135, 137

R

radioallergosorbent test (RAST)   46, 101-103

radiography   46

ragweed   98

retinal artery occlusion   127

rhinitis   25, 41, 91, 118
   allergic   10, 36, 94, 98, 100, 101

rhinitis medicamentosa   25, 91, 92, 96

Rhinocort®   95

rhinorrhea   46, 97, 98, 116

rhinoscopy   17, 41

rhinoviruses   26, 30, 36

Rhizopus   29, 74, 77

Rocephin®   87

S

saline nasal drops   129

saline nasal spray   92-96, 123

scarring   113, 131

scars   113

scintillation counter   102

sclerosis   65

sedimentation rate   128

seizure   119

Seldane-D®   100

Seldane®   99

Semprex™-D   100

senile rhinorrhea   25

sepsis   72, 74, 127

septa   9, 14

septal perforation   96

septated hyphae   76

septicemia   73

septoplasty   107

Septra®   83

serial end-point titration (SET)   101

serous glands   48

serum immunoglobulin levels   45

sinus cavities   19, 23

sinus opacification   67, 75

sinus ostia   19-21

sinus puncture   44

sinus surgery   120, 124

sinus thrombosis   126, 127

Sinuses

    anterior sinus drainage
        system   18

    paranasal sinuses   12, 13,
        16, 17, 19, 21, 47, 48, 51,
        67, 68, 117

        ethmoid   12-14, 16, 18,
            20, 21, 41, 42, 46, 48, 49,
            52, 57, 78, 91, 107, 110,
            111, 125, 131

        frontal   12-16, 18, 20, 42,
            46, 48-50, 54, 57, 78,
            107, 108, 110, 116, 117,
            131

        maxillary   12-14, 16, 18,
            20, 21, 27, 36, 41, 42, 46,
            48, 49, 57, 67, 75, 78,
            107, 108, 110, 111, 116,
            117, 131

        sphenoid   12, 13, 16, 20,
            46, 48, 50, 57, 65, 78,
            111, 131

Sinusitis   6, 7, 9

    acute   5, 8, 26, 28, 29, 36,
        37, 40, 57, 59, 66, 92-94,
        96, 121, 128

    Aspergillus   75

    bacterial   10, 19, 25, 26, 37,
        72, 78, 81, 83-86, 89, 90

    chronic   5, 7- 9, 28, 29, 36,
        40, 44-47, 51, 60, 91,
        94-97, 108, 109, 116,
        119, 120, 122, 135, 137

    definition of   7

    frontal   38, 53

    fungal   10, 30, 60, 72, 74

    in the elderly   10

    intracranial complications
        of   132

    maxillary   11, 37, 53, 73

    medical cost of   7

    nosocomial   38, 72, 74, 78

      bacterial   73

    orbital complications
        of   125, 126

    pansinusitis   110, 111

    pathophysiology of   5

    prevalence of   7

    recurrent   5, 7, 46, 60

    recurrent acute   8, 63, 94,
        109, 116, 120, 121

    rhinosinusitis   37, 79, 97,
        99, 102, 109

    sinus surgical procedures   8

    sphenoid   38, 53

    subacute   8

    surgical management
        of   106

    surgical procedures for
      Caldwell-Luc opera-
        tion   106

      external
       ethmoidectomy   106

      frontoethmoidectomy   106

      intranasal
       ethmoidectomy   106

      transnasal
       ethmoidectomy   106

    viral rhinosinusitis   85, 89

skin end-point titration
  (SET)   102, 103

sleep apnea   69

smoking   10

smoking addiction   9

sneezing   9, 46, 96-98, 100

sore throat   40

sparfloxacin (Zagam®)   82, 83, 85-87

spasm   126, 127

sperm motility   45

sphenoethmoid recess   16, 18, 42-44, 111

Sporanox®   30, 76

staphylococci   78, 79

Staphylococcus aureus   26, 28, 30, 73, 79, 83, 88, 94, 128, 132

strenuous sports   135

streptococci   29

Streptococcus pneumoniae   9, 10, 27, 28, 30, 45, 78, 81, 82, 84, 88, 89, 92, 94, 128

subdural abscess   132

subperiosteal abscess   126, 127, 130, 131

Surgery
   arthroscopic surgery   112
   endoscopic joint surgery   112
   endoscopic sinus surgery   112
   nasal polyp surgery   112
   temporomandibular joint surgery   112

surgery   120-122, 127, 129

surgical débridement   76, 77

sweat chloride   45

sweat chloride testing   46

swelling   41, 43, 59

synechiae   113, 118, 123

T

terfenadine (Seldane®)   99

tetracaine (Pontocaine®)   43

tetracycline   84

thrombophlebitis   125

thromboxanes   100

tobacco smoke   9

Tornwaldt's cyst   56

torus tubarius   44

tranquilizers   102

transillumination   38, 44, 58

trauma   36, 41, 72, 131

trees   98

trephination   130

triamcinolone acetonide (Nasacort®)   95

trimethoprim/sulfamethoxazole (Bactrim™, Septra®)   82, 83, 85, 87, 88, 90

tripelennamine (PBZ®)   99

tumors   25, 36, 41, 91, 118

turbinate hypertrophy   91

turbinates   17, 21, 37, 55, 111, 112
   inferior   17, 43, 45
   middle   17, 18, 43, 45
   superior   17, 43
   supreme turbinate   17

turbinectomy   111, 113

U

ultrasonography (US)   57

uncinate process   18, 20, 43, 66, 110

upper respiratory tract infection (URI)   8, 9, 36, 37, 41, 45, 91, 118, 119

V

Valsalva's maneuver   10

Vancenase®   95

vancomycin (Vancocin®)   87, 88, 90

vasoconstriction   100

vasomotor rhinitis   36

venous sinus thrombosis   132

Vibramycin®   83

voice resonance   12, 13

W

walking   135

Waters' projection   59

watery eyes   97

Wegener's granulomatosis   45, 91

white blood cell (WBC)   129

X

x-rays   5, 12, 14, 15, 45, 46, 53, 54, 68, 128

xenon   69

Xylocaine®   43

Z

Zagam®   83

zinc   85

Zithromax®   83

zygomycosis   75, 77

Zyrtec®   99

NOTES

NOTES

NOTES

NOTES

NOTES

NOTES

NOTES

NOTES

NOTES

NOTES